HEALTH JOURNEY
Your Personal Road Map for Vibrant Living & Youthful Aging

Packed with the latest information about
Nutrition
Water
Going Green
Genetically Modified Organisms
Food Combining
Portion Control
Juice Fasting
Transitioning to Raw Foods
Raw Food Preparation
Simple Recipes
Exercise for All Ages
Making Lifestyle Changes
Recommendations for Better Health

LILLIAN R. BUTLER
EDDIE D. ROBINSON

HEALTH JOURNEY
Your Personal Road Map for Vibrant Living and Youthful Aging

Raw Soul
348 W. 145th Street
New York, NY 10039
Email: rawsoul@rawsoul.com
Website: www.rawsoul.com

Copyright 2007, 2008 Labor of Love Productions, LLC

All rights reserved. No part of this material may be reproduced in any form or by any means without written permission from the publisher.

The information contained in this book is not meant as a substitute for medical advice. Its intention is solely informational and educational. Please consult a medical or health professional should the need for one be indicated.

Published by
Labor of Love Productions, LLC
P. O. Box 7135
New York, NY 10150
212-491-5859

ISBN 978-0-9814634-0-7

Cover design by Premium Image Makers
www.pimnyc.com, 212-281-6200

DEDICATION

This book is dedicated in loving memory of my mother, Bernadine Butler, whose untimely death led me to seek the answers to health and healing.

SAYING GOODBYE AND HELLO

Saying goodbye and letting go
Is hard to do I know
But saying goodbye and letting go
Is the only way to say hello

Yvonne M. Jenkins

CONTENTS

ACKNOWLEDGEMENTS viii

FOREWARD ix

INTRODUCTION xi

1   GOOD NUTRITION 17
    Free Radicals 17
    Antioxidants 18
    Carbohydrates 19
    Proteins 20
    Fats 23
    Vitamins 25
    Minerals 27
    Phytonutrients 30
    Water 31
    Whole Foods 37
    Plant-based Food Guide Pyramid 42
    Recommendations for Better Health 43

2   FOODS TO AVOID FOR OPTIMUM HEALTH 45
    Processed Foods 45
    Animal-Based Foods 48
    Cooked Foods 50
    Genetically Modified Organisms 51
    Canola Oil 54
    Soy Products 55
    Recommendations for Better Health 57

3	**GOING GREEN**	59
	The Greenhouse Effect	59
	Holes in the Ozone Layer	60
	Air Pollution and Acid Rain	60
	Water Pollution	61
	Chemical Toxins	61
	Modern Living	62
	Too Much Trash	62
	Going Green Guidelines	63
	Support Sustainable Practices	65
	Buy and Eat Locally Grown Foods	65
	Eat Foods in Season	65
	Buy Organically Grown Produce	66
	Recommendations for Better Health	68
4	**CULTIVATING GOOD HABITS**	69
	Eat Just Enough	69
	What Constitutes A Serving?	72
	Proper Food Combining	73
	Food Combining Guidelines	74
	Length of Time Foods Stay in the Stomach	75
	Alkaline-Forming Foods	76
	Juicing	77
	Juicing Guidelines	78
	Juice Fasting	79
	Colon Care	81
	Recommendations for Better Health	84
5	**ADOPTING A PLANT-BASED DIET**	85
	Raw and Living Foods	86
	Pantry	94
	Setting Up A Raw Kitchen	96
	The Six Tastes	101
	Meal Planning	102
	Food Preparation Guidelines	103

6 RECIPES	**105**
Soaking and Sprouting	105
Beverages	108
Sauces	112
Nut and Seed Cheese	114
Soups	115
Salads	117
Salad Dressings	121
Pâtés	123
Side Dishes	125
Main Dishes	128
Bread, Fritters and Pancakes	134
Desserts	136
Recommendations for Better Health	142
7 LIFESTYLE	**143**
A Positive Attitude	143
Breathing	144
Relaxation	145
Sleep	146
Meditation	146
Exercise	147
Recommendations for Better Health	149
BIBLIOGRAPHY	**151**
AFTERWARD	**153**

ACKNOWLEDGEMENTS

Thank you to all of our customers, students, friends and family whose repeated requests motivated us to write this book. To the teachers and volunteers at the Ann Wigmore Institute and Optimum Health Institute for your knowledge, guidance and inspiration.

To our many customers who sing our praises. We appreciate you and thank you from the bottom of our hearts. To Ellen Benoit, Max Cargill, Ohbeeb Cavalcante, and Cookie WInborn who gave generously of your time and expertise in proofreading this book over and over again.

To our dedicated staff at Raw Soul whose commitment and loving spirit have contributed greatly to the completion of this book.

To all of you who are part of the raw and living foods movement. Without your commitment and struggle, none of this would be possible.

To the pioneers of this movement for your courage, commitment and inspiration.

And ultimately to the universal spirit for mentoring us and guiding us on this path of enlightenment!

FOREWARD

**DR. ROBERT WOODBINE, N.D., M.Ac.O.M., L.Ac.
President, San Bao Holistic Care**

The American medical system is in crisis and the people who depend on it for succor are actively seeking alternatives. It is a system that operates in a society touted to be the richest and most technologically advanced in the world. Yet, the World Health Organization ranks American healthcare an average of fifteenth out of the twenty-five industrialized nations.

Nearly one million Americans die annually, at a cost of over $282 Billion due to iatrogenic causes. These are deaths that are induced inadvertently by a physician or surgeon or drug error, or by medical treatment or diagnostic procedure. After heart disease and cancer, the third leading cause of death in America is the medical care system itself. This is, at minimum, frightening and appalling.

As a Cartesian, disease-based model of care that promotes dependency on pharmaceutical or surgical intervention, traditional American medicine fails to focus on prevention and wellness. It is not a patient-centered or community focused system. As a whole, it is part of the cultural mindset driven by the same forces that doggedly refute the veracity of global warming, pollute our air, water, soil and food supply, denigrate the poor, and bow before the altar of consumerism.

This book offers a blueprint for change that strikes at the core of this problem. More than an excellent primer on nutrition, water, food combining, and wonderful recipes, it is a prescription for a revolution. A revolution of consciousness to acknowledge our intrinsic capacity for optimal wellness through "...accepting responsibility for our health and the choices we make." And what makes this book invaluable is the focus and emphasis on the importance of cultivating family, and thus community, as well as supporting sustainable farming to promote self-sufficiency.

This book is one more example of Lillian and Eddie's deep commitment to humanity to break the ties and lies that bind the mind from liberation.

INTRODUCTION

Good health is your right! But changing lifelong habits and patterns is not easy. It requires focused energy, freeing the mind of stagnant beliefs, opening the heart to love and kindness, and developing intuition. Some of us are more motivated than others. Certainly an illness or disease gives us motivation to make changes. Please don't wait until you're in a health crisis to start making changes. Make changes now to avoid a health crisis in the future.

We are advocating a healing lifestyle, not a diet. Obviously if you are reading this book, you have made some decisions about improving your health. In order to do that, you must begin by omitting certain foods that are detrimental to your health. These foods include meat, dairy, fried foods, refined foods (sugar, salt, white flour), and packaged foods. Not only are these foods detrimental to your health, but they accelerate aging.

Hand-in-hand with these detrimental foods are bad habits such as smoking, drinking and drugging, that must be eliminated. Not even moderate health can be realized while saturating your body with these poisons.

Equally important are stressful situations and people in your life. It is time to take a good hard look at all of these factors and begin to make changes. Surround yourself with positive, like-minded people. You will be amazed at how good you feel in a short period of time. The body has the ability to heal itself, particularly when placed in the right environment.

You deserve vital health. Give yourself the opportunity to experience life without illness, disease, pain and suffering. In a very short period of time you will experience increased energy, better sleep, less stress and emotional eating. Through the intake of living foods and through juice fasting, you will begin to deal with emotions that you have been stuffing for many years. Our emotions, positive and negative, have deep connections to food. When one begins to detoxify from food and those toxins enter the bloodstream, so do those emotions that were never dealt with and consequently have been making you ill. As these emotions present themselves, allow yourself to feel them, and get to the root of the situation. Don't be afraid to feel. Most of us don't want to feel negative emotions, so we "stuff" them with food. But just like toxic food, negative emotions make us ill.

Please read this book completely. We have painstakingly selected recipes that are nutritious and easy to prepare. Other than a blender and maybe a food processor, you will not need to purchase any expensive equipment. Stop eating out so much and get in the kitchen and prepare food for yourself and your family. It is the only way to ensure you are getting a healthy, balanced meal.

When you eat at various restaurants, you are putting your health in the hands of the person making the food. Do you know if they practice proper hygiene? What is their state of mind? Are they upset, sad, angry, or perhaps indifferent? Do they love what they are doing, or is it just a job? Is the food fresh or did they open a can and doctor up the ingredients? Is the food made with love? You have no way of knowing.

Don't get me wrong, eating out from time to time can and should be enjoyed, but when it becomes a way of life, one must question the quality of life. When you do eat out, get to know the proprietor and employees. Eat at places where you know the food is prepared with love, using high-quality fresh ingredients by people who care about you. Select a few good places and frequent them from time to time.

Don't be bashful about asking for something that is not on the menu. Ask for what you want. Most chefs like a challenge. Requesting a vegetarian or raw dish is usually not too difficult.

Sit down and experience a delicious home-prepared meal with your family and friends. The best memories of my childhood are helping my mother prepare food, and sitting at the table eating with my six brothers and sisters. No matter what else we were doing, we all ate dinner together, and what a good time we had. We would pray, sing, laugh, and cry right at the dinner table. Although we were stuffing ourselves, it was emotionally cleansing!

Many of our dinner guests included extended family members such as neighbors, friends, and family. If you were hungry, you could dine at our table. This provided an important social structure to our community. The elderly, sick and lonely were provided for and taken care of. If you weren't seen in the neighborhood, someone would knock on your door to make sure you were alright. This is a true community.

However, in New York City, where we live, most people don't know their neighbors. What's more, when they see them they don't speak, and do not want to be bothered with them knocking on their door. When people want to get together they invite you to meet at a restaurant. Rarely are you invited to dinner at someone's home. This is why we are so disconnected from one another. Reach out to your neighbors and at the very least say "hello." Take an interest in the elderly. See how you can make their lives easier. Invite your neighbors, friends, and family over for a home-cooked meal. It doesn't have to be something elaborate. Dining at someone's home makes the experience personal and even intimate. One can really relax and enjoy the good food and great company.

My path began when I accompanied my friend, Audrey, to the Ann Wigmore Institute in Puerto Rico. There I was introduced to fresh wheat grass juice, sprouting, blended soups, and the taking of enemas. It was very strange to me in the beginning, but I felt so good, and had so much energy after a few days, I knew I had to stick with it. That was 8 years ago! Learning about living foods changed my life completely.

Eddie and I are not chefs by trade, and never in a million years did we think that we would own a restaurant. But we love it! We are so blessed to be able to share our love with the world by providing good healthy food. We have included recipes taken from our menus and classes at Raw Soul Restaurant in New

York City. These recipes have been thoroughly developed, tested and refined. Magic happens when you make food everyday. You refine your skills, simplify recipes, develop creativity (oftentimes through so-called "mistakes"), and learn about yourself. Preparing food requires caring, time, organization, knowledge, skill, patience, and creativity. In other words, love! No half measures! Take the time and care to prepare your meals and they will always turn out great. Try out new recipes on co-workers, neighbors, friends, family!

The information offered in this book is taken from our personal experiences, along with the latest research and nutritional information regarding health and longevity. Use this book as a resource for maintaining and regaining a high level of health. The procedures are offered as tools to assist you in developing a personal health regime.

You have made the decision to choose health. Back it up with commitment and action. Stick with it. Be patient and kind to yourself and you will experience health at a level you never thought possible!

Lillian R. Butler

1

GOOD NUTRITION
THE FOUNDATION OF A
BALANCED DIET

Why do we eat? We eat to give the body fuel. Food is the body's fuel. Just as there are different qualities of fuel for automobiles (leaded, unleaded, premium, super premium), there are different qualities of fuel for our bodies (processed foods, whole foods). We must begin with putting good food (fuel) into our bodies for optimum performance.

Poor quality foods are difficult to digest, absorb, and eliminate. They deplete the body of vitamins and minerals, increase the body's toxic load, increase blood sugar, raise cholesterol levels, create free radicals, and lead to nutritional imbalances and malnutrition.

FREE RADICALS are oxygen molecules found in a cell that has lost an electron and become unstable. To heal itself it steals electrons from healthy cells, creating more free radicals. Free radicals are generated through a variety of activities, including the conversion of food into energy, air pollution, sun damage, cigarette smoke, alcohol, stress, long term use of certain medications, x-rays, improperly combined foods, and grilled, fried, and fast foods. The results of free radical damage include premature aging, poor health, stroke, and the onset of diseases such as cancer, arthritis, diabetes, arteriosclerosis, and senility.

Health Journey

Poor quality foods are foods made with white flour (bread, pasta, and baked goods), white sugar, high fructose corn syrup, cooked grains, fried foods, white rice, potatoes, meat, dairy, and all refined and processed foods such as packaged and canned foods that contain preservatives.

Nutrient-dense foods are easy to digest, absorb and eliminate. They flood the body with natural vitamins and minerals heal free radical damage to the cells, increase energy, balance blood sugar, and lower cholesterol.

Nutrient-dense foods include fruits, leafy greens, vegetables, whole grains, nuts and seeds.

ANTIOXIDANTS are our body's superheroes, as they help neutralize free radicals before they cause tissue and cellular damage. Our bodies manufacture enzyme antioxidants known as superoxide dismutase (SOD), glutathione, peroxidase and catalase. Antioxidants derived from food are Vitamins A, C, E, and beta carotene, and the minerals zinc, copper, selenium, and manganese. Food-derived and enzyme antioxidants work as a team to effectively fight free radicals. If we are deficient in any of these vitamins and minerals, our body's ability to neutralize free radicals is impaired.

Other antioxidants include the amino acids cysteine, methionine and lysine. In addition to fighting free radicals, they perform a number of functions such as guarding against cirrhosis of the liver, removing toxins and metals from the system, regenerating tissue, and boosting the immune system.

Antioxidants lycopene, lutein, and carotenoids are found in the skin of fruits and vegetables. Not only do they fight free radicals, but they reduce the risk of certain cancers. (See Phytonutrients on page 30 for further discussion).

A balanced diet consists of a wide variety and ample amounts of nutrient dense foods to support good health. Nutrients provide energy, promote the growth and maintenance of the body, and/or regulate body processes. Nutrients consist of carbohydrates, proteins, fats, vitamins, minerals, and water. All of these play important roles in a well-balanced diet.

CARBOHYDRATES are a large class of nutrients, including sugars, starches, and fibers. Their function in the body is to provide energy. All carbohydrates are broken down into simple sugars (glucose).

Unrefined simple carbohydrates are found in natural fruits with seeds. Select fruits that are richly mineralized and low in sugar such as apples, pears, berries of all kinds, citrus fruits, mangoes, melons and papayas.

High-quality complex carbohydrates are found in whole grains, vegetables, and sprouted legumes (such as lentils). Good sources are brussels sprouts, collard greens, green beans, cauliflower, and red and yellow bell peppers (green bell peppers are unripe peppers and should be avoided.) They are loaded with fiber, vitamins, minerals and phytonutrients that **heal free radical damage** to the cells and fight cancer.

Starch is found in breads, breakfast cereals, pastas, potatoes, beans and vegetables. Sweet potatoes, yams, corn, rutabagas, turnips, sprouted grains and beans are good starch choices.

Health Journey

Fiber is obtained only from plant sources. It cannot be broken down or digested and is therefore useful in sucking up toxic chemicals, fats, cholesterol and heavy metals and escorting them out of the body. Fiber reduces the risk of heart disease, improves digestion, absorption and elimination, stabilizes blood pressure and sugar, and aids in weight loss.

There are two types: 1) Soluble--dissolves in water. Found in apples, squash, strawberries, blueberries, bran, lentils, peas, beans and green beans; 2) Insoluble–found in whole grains, all nuts and seeds, carrots, cucumbers, celery, and zucchini. Flax seeds contain insoluble and soluble fiber.

PROTEINS are molecular compounds that are integral to the life and function of every living cell. Proteins build muscle, strengthen tissues, and repair cells. Enzymes, hormones, and genes are made up of proteins. Amino acids are the building blocks of proteins. Most amino acids are manufactured by our body, but there are nine that must be obtained from dietary sources. These are known as essential amino acids and include Tryptophan, Threonine, Isoleucine, Leucine, Lysine, Methionine and Cystine, Phenylalanine and Tyrosine, Valine and Histidine..

Animal protein is not the best source of protein. The protein found in animal muscle tissue is very concentrated and difficult to absorb, putting a burden on the kidneys and the liver. The amount of protein we need has been greatly exaggerated. To calculate how many grams of protein you need daily, multiply your weight in pounds by 0.36 grams (i.e., if you weigh 150 pounds, multiply your weight by 0.36 grams protein per pound = 54 grams of protein you need daily).

Good Nutrition

Plant proteins found in whole grains, fresh grass juices, algaes, green leafy vegetables, legumes, nuts, seeds and sprouts can sufficiently supply the body's protein needs without adding a significant amount of calories and raising cholesterol levels. Plant proteins are easy to digest and assimilate and offer an abundance of vitamins, minerals and fiber.

Sources of complete plant proteins include grass juices, algaes, quinoa and hemp seeds.

Leafy greens and whole grains are carbohydrates that contain a good amount of protein. Although their amino acid profile is incomplete, eating a variety of protein-rich foods in large amounts will form complete proteins. Green leafy vegetables include collard greens, kale, mustard greens, turnip greens, cabbage, arugula, dandelion, spinach, sorrel, Swiss chard, and watercress. Whole grains include amaranth, barley, buckwheat, corn, kamut, millet, quinoa, rye, spelt, wheat and wild rice.

Legumes, nuts and seeds are protein foods that offer the highest amount of proteins. Legumes include lentils, chickpeas, adzuki beans, and other beans of all kinds.

Nuts include almonds, walnuts, hazelnuts, Brazil nuts, pecans, macadamia nuts and pine nuts.

Seeds include chia seeds, flaxseeds, hemp seeds, sunflower seeds and pumpkin seeds.

Sprouts include sprouted grains, legumes and seeds mentioned above, and vegetable sprouts such as alfalfa, broccoli, cabbage, clover, fenugreek and radish.

Health Journey

The following chart lists plant foods that offer a significant amount of protein.

Grains	Unit	Grams Protein	Grams Fat
Buckwheat (raw)	1 cup	24	2
Buckwheat (cooked)	1 cup	7	1
Corn (raw)	1 cup	16	8
Corn (cooked)	1 cup	4	1
Millet (raw)	1 cup	22	8
Millet (cooked)	1 cup	6	2
Quinoa (raw)	1 cup	24	2
Quinoa (cooked)	1 cup	7	1
Legumes	**Unit**	**Grams Protein**	**Grams Fat**
Chickpeas (raw)	1 cup	39	12
Chickpeas (cooked)	1 cup	15	11
Lentils (raw)	1 cup	50	2
Lentils (cooked)	1 cup	18	1
Nuts and Seeds	**Unit**	**Grams Protein**	**Grams Fat**
Brazil Nuts	1 cup	20	48
Cashews	1 cup	20	63
Flax Seeds (whole)	1 cup	31	71
Hazelnuts (Filberts)	1 cup	11	46
Hemp Seeds	½ cup	30	27
Macadamia Nuts	½ cup	5 ½	51
Pecans	1 cup	10	78
Pine Nuts	½ cup	9	46
Pistachios	1 cup.	25	55
Pumpkin Seeds	1 cup	12	12
Sesame Seeds	½ cup	13	36
Sunflower Seeds (hulled)	1 cup	24	63
Walnuts	1 cup	18	76

These numbers are based on raw grains, legumes, nuts and seeds that have **not** been soaked and sprouted. When foods are soaked and sprouted their volume and nutritional content is increased. Notice that cooked grains and legumes have less protein.

The fats in nuts and seeds are primarily heart-healthy monounsaturated and polyunsaturated. Studies reveal that consuming a handful of nuts per day results in a drop of approximately 50% in the risk of heart disease by lowering cholesterol levels.

FATS are a group of fatty substances, including triglycerides and cholesterol that are soluble in fat, not water. The arrangement of hydrogen determines if a fat is saturated, monounsaturated, or polyunsaturated. Fats are broken down into fatty acids.

Fats are necessary for the absorption of the fat-soluble vitamins A, D, E, and K. Good fats are necessary for normal function and development of the brain. They lubricate the joints, thereby aiding in the prevention of arthritis, produce energy and help to keep us warm.

Saturated Fats consist of two groups of fats–medium and long–chain and each acts differently in the body. Long chain saturates are found primarily in animal products like fat from meat, butter, cheese, and other milk products. These fats raise levels of LDL (bad) cholesterol and lower levels of HDL (good) cholesterol. They also contribute to colon and prostate cancers. Medium-chain saturates from plant sources such as coconuts are easily digested and do not clog arteries. Coconut oil is naturally saturated and never needs to be hydrogenated (the process that changes fat from liquid to solid, thereby creating Trans Fatty Acids).

Monounsaturated Fats found in olives, avocados and nuts (almonds, cashews, hazelnuts macadamia nuts, pecans and pistachio nuts) help lower damaging LDL cholesterol levels. They also contain antioxidants that combat clogging of the arteries and chronic diseases, including cancer.

Polyunsaturated Fats are found primarily in corn oil, hemp seeds, pumpkin seeds, sesame seeds, sunflower seeds and walnuts. Polyunsaturated fats help lower LDL cholesterol levels.

Essential Fatty Acids (EFAs), known as Omega-3 and Omega-6 fatty acids help reduce the risk of heart disease, diabetes II and stroke, support the immune system, guard against viral infections, help improve brain function, lower blood pressure, regulate hormone levels, and are beneficial to healthy hair, skin and nails.

EFAs must be obtained from dietary sources. Ideally you want one food source that contains Omega-3 and Omega-6 fatty acids in a 2:1 ratio such as flaxseeds, hemp seeds, pumpkin seeds, walnuts, evening primrose oil, black currant oil and sea vegetables.

Oils are sensitive to heat, light and oxygen. Exposure to these elements during or after processing oxidizes the oil causing it to go rancid. Rancid oils are indigestible and cannot be utilized by the body. Heating oil at high temperatures also causes free radical damage to the cells which accelerates aging.

Good Nutrition

VITAMINS are organic nutrients without calories. They are essential in regulating body processes, maintenance, growth and reproduction. Vitamins A, D, E and K are fat soluble and stay in the body longer. All other vitamins–the B-complex group and Vitamin C–are water soluble, and are eliminated from the body through urine and perspiration. Water soluble vitamins stay in the body for four days at the most and must be replenished frequently. Let's take a look at the water soluble vitamins, their function and vegetarian food sources.

Vitamin B Complex consists of 11 components that have important functions in the body, and are all inter-related:

Vitamin B1 (Thiamine) facilitates the conversion of sugar and starch into energy. Best food sources are sea vegetables (dulse, hijiki) and yellow, red and green vegetables.

Vitamin B2 (Riboflavin) provides cells with fuel and air, and mobilizes and converts proteins, fats and carbohydrates to energy and structural components. Food sources include hijiki, nutritional yeast, nuts, legumes, leafy green vegetables and whole grains.

Vitamin B3 (Niacin) helps synthesize sex hormones, cortisone, insulin and thyroxine. It aids in metabolizing fats, lowering cholesterol and improving blood circulation. Food sources include kelp, avocados, dates, figs, prunes, legumes and whole grains.

Vitamin B5 (Pantothenic Acid) stimulates the adrenal glands to produce the necessary stress hormones. Food sources include kelp, whole grains, green vegetables, potatoes, nuts and nutritional yeast.

Health Journey

Vitamin B6 (Pyridoxine) strengthens the immune system, is a natural diuretic, and alleviates nausea. Food sources include avocados, cabbage, kelp and walnuts.

Vitamin B12 (Cobalamin) forms and regenerates red blood cells, increases energy, and improves concentration. A high percentage of meat eaters and vegetarians are deficient in Vitamin B12. It is found in small amounts in kelp, kombu, laver, Irish moss, algaes and wheat grass juice. Have your B12 levels tested to determine if supplementation is necessary.

Folic Acid (Vitamin M) synthesizes proteins and genetic materials DNA and RNA, and protects against intestinal parasites and food poisoning. Food sources include green leafy vegetables, carrots, cantaloupe, apricots, pumpkin, avocado, beans, whole grains, broccoli and cabbage.

Biotin (Vitamin H) aids in keeping hair from turning gray and the prevention of baldness and alleviates eczema and dermatitis. Food sources include romaine lettuce, carrots, Swiss chard, cauliflower and peas.

Inositol helps lower cholesterol levels, promotes healthy hair, skin and nails, and helps prevent eczema. Food sources include cantaloupe, grapefruit, oranges, limes, cabbage, raisins, beans and wheat germ.

Choline helps stimulate memory and thought processes, and aids the liver in eliminating drugs and poisons from your system. Food sources include seed oils such as flax and grape seed, whole grains, cereals, legumes and green leafy vegetables.

Good Nutrition

Para-Aminobenzoic Acid (PABA) maintains healthy skin and hair, delays wrinkles, and helps restore natural color. Food sources include molasses, whole grains and wheat germ.

Vitamin C is vital to the overall structural and functional integrity of muscles, bones, teeth, skin, and connective tissues. It is necessary for general growth of body cells, fighting infection and reducing stress. Food sources include hijiki, wakame, kelp, sesame seeds, broccoli and cabbage.

MINERALS are required by the body in small amounts and do not provide energy. The body does not manufacture minerals, so they must be obtained through diet. They are naturally occurring elements found in the earth. They are passed from the soil to the plants. We in turn obtain the minerals from the plants. Some minerals, such as calcium and phosphorous become part of the body's structure in the bones and teeth. Minerals are broken up into two groups: 1) macro or bulk, those your body uses in large amounts, and 2) trace, those needed in small amounts.

Bulk Minerals

Calcium is essential for bone, tooth, and muscular development, as well as metabolic processes in the body. Calcium can help lower blood pressure and prevent colon cancer, heart disease, and osteoporosis. For the body to properly use calcium, phosphorus and magnesium must combine with calcium in 1:1 and 2:1 ratios, respectively. Food sources include sea vegetables: arame, hijiki, kelp, kombu, Irish moss, and wakame; blackstrap molasses, sesame seeds, leafy green vegetables, cabbage and walnuts. Calcium absorption is aided by Vitamin D, so be sure to get lots of sunshine!

Phosphorus is needed for bone strength, energy, and the metabolism of fats, proteins and carbohydrates. It is abundant in the body. Too much can decrease calcium absorption. Be aware of foods preserved with phosphorous. Food sources include legumes, whole grains, nuts and seeds.

Magnesium is essential to effective nerve, muscle, and bone functioning. It helps fight kidney stones, diabetes and osteoporosis. Food sources include hijiki, wakame, Irish moss, blackstrap molasses, unmilled grains, almonds, figs, nuts, seeds, and dark green vegetables.

Potassium works inside the cells to regulate fluid balance and normalize heart rhythms. Helps dispose of waste and reduce blood pressure. Food sources include citrus fruits, cantaloupe, dried apricots, avocado, bananas, all green leafy vegetables, broccoli, lima beans, legumes and potatoes.

Sodium works with potassium to help maintain the body's fluid balance. Most of us get too much sodium from unnatural sources such as table salt, canned foods, luncheon meats, frankfurters, salt-cured meats, ketchup, soy sauce, mustard and junk food. Natural food sources include celery, sea vegetables, olives, sea salt, carrots and beets.

Trace minerals are needed in small amounts but are essential. These minerals include chlorine, chromium, copper, iodine, iron, manganese, molybdenum, selenium, and zinc. If you include a variety of fruits, sea vegetables, leafy green vegetables, whole grains,

Good Nutrition

nuts, and seeds in your daily diet, you will more than likely get an adequate amount of these minerals in your diet. There is one, however, that needs pointing out:

Iron is essential in bringing oxygen to the cells. It is necessary for the production of hemoglobin in the red blood cells and the production of enzymes for energy. It helps strengthen the immune cells, and is important for absorption and utilization of all the B vitamins.

Women of child-bearing age, teenagers, children, some infants and the elderly are commonly deficient in iron.

Iron is found in two forms—heme, found in flesh foods (meat, poultry, and fish) and non-heme, found in vegetables. Absorption of dietary iron is influenced primarily by the body's need for iron, how much iron is stored in the body, and dietary factors. Tannins found in tea, polyphenols found in coffee, phytates found in whole grains, bran, and soy products, and oxalates found in spinach, rhubarb, and chocolate inhibit iron absorption. Soaking and sprouting whole grains such as buckwheat, amaranth, and millet will eliminate phytates.

Hydrochloric Acid (HCl) and Vitamin C aid in the absorption of non-heme iron. The presence of acidic foods such as orange, lemon and lime juice, and apple cider vinegar help stimulate HCl production and enhance non-heme iron absorption. High vitamin C foods include red bell peppers, celery, lemon and lime.

The best plant-based food sources of iron include leafy greens such as collards, kale, mustards, spinach Swiss chard and turnips; Jerusalem artichokes, onions, asparagus, Burdock root, blackberries, cherries, lettuce, nettles and parsley.

Health Journey

PHYTONUTRIENTS are organic compounds, not nutrients, found in the green, red, yellow, orange or blue of fruits and vegetables and grains. Scientists are just now discovering the role these substances play in preventing disease, enhancing memory and increasing one's life span. Phytonutrients can have a profound impact on our health because they function as antioxidants.

Cruciferous vegetables contain vital cancer-fighting phytonutrients. They include broccoli, bok choy, brussels sprouts, cabbage, cauliflower, collards, daikon, kale, napa cabbage, radishes, rutabagas, turnips and watercress.

Berries of all kinds (particularly goji, and açai), citrus fruits (including pomegranates), grapes and grape seeds are phytonutrients known as bioflavonoids. Bioflavonoids help the function of Vitamin C in the body. This and their antioxidant properties make them essential in optimizing health and alleviating diseases caused by aging.

Carrots, celery, onions, garlic, peppers, tomatoes, watermelon, green tea, and turmeric are phytonutrients that are high in antioxidants (vitamins, A, C, E, and selenium), and helpful in lowering cholesterol and blood pressure, fighting tooth decay, and reducing the risk of heart disease, cancer and cataracts.

Phytoestrogens (isoflavones) are a group of chemicals found in plant foods such as beans, seeds, and grains that mimic the hormone estrogen. Soy products have some of the highest levels of phytoestrogens, Recent scientific research suggests that high doses of soy phytoestrogens increase the risk of breast cancer. See page 55 for more information.

WATER

Water ranks second only to oxygen as essential to life. Water plays a vital role in all bodily processes and makes up just over half of the body's weight.

There are many **benefits** to drinking water: it aids in weight loss, keeps the bowels moving, prevents dehydration, flushes toxins out of vital organs, carries nutrients to cells, particularly the brain, prevents kidney stone formation, moistens air passages, sinuses and lungs, and gives you a clear complexion.

We have a water pollution problem. Tap water can contain countless harmful substances, including arsenic, lead, herbicides, parasites, sulfates, pesticides, mercury, aluminum, radon, chlorine, and fluoride. Many local municipalities add chlorine and fluoride to the drinking water.

Chlorine in the water you drink, bathe and swim in can cause massive scarring of the arteries, which leads to clogged arteries, arteriosclerosis, and heart disease.

Fluoride has been linked to serious and massive health problems. Research reveals that even small amounts can damage the immune system, inhibit the action of enzymes, create arthritic conditions or encourage pre-existing ones, and cause dental fluorosis in children. Permanent visible signs of dental fluorosis are white spots, staining and chalky and brittle tooth enamel.

Have your drinking water tested by your local health department to determine what's in it. Once you know, I recommend purchasing a water filtration system for your home. At the very least purchase a good filter for your kitchen sink and shower. Look for a system that uses both activated carbon and reverse osmosis to filter all chemical contaminants. The skin is the largest detoxification organ and absorbs toxins. Showering and bathing in tap water is the equivalent of drinking it.

Bottled water is at best a temporary solution. Think of all the ways you use water. For drinking, washing hands, bathing, washing produce, cooking, ice cubes, cooling off. It can become very expensive and impractical to use bottled water for all of these uses. Besides, the safety of bottled water is questionable. Much bottled water is tap water with a fancy label.

What Type of Water to Drink?

Spring water that has been charged with nature's energy for hundreds of years and bottled at the source is the best drinking water. Make sure your spring water is low in minerals and free from pollutants such as nitrates. Most spring water found in the supermarket has been carbonated by adding artificial nitrogen and extracting natural hydrogen. Natural artesian Fiji water from the Fiji Islands contains healthy forms of colloidal silica and has a slightly alkaline pH of 7.5.

Mineral water that is bottled has been processed and its natural electromagnetic frequencies and vibration patterns are altered. In general, the minerals in water are too coarse to be absorbed by our bodies.

Distillation of water produces the purest water, but the geometric structure of the water is destroyed, making it acidic, and causing it to bind with other elements. For this reason never buy distilled water in plastic bottles.

Reverse osmosis removes nearly all pollutants, but negative vibration patterns are left from the toxins. Add quartz crystals to revitalize the water allowing them to soak in the water for 8 hours.

How Much Water to Drink?

Most of us do not drink enough water. We lose water through breathing, perspiration, urine and bowel movements. We must replenish this water in order for our bodies to function properly. Beverages and food containing water make up 20% of your fluid intake. The remaining 80% must come from drinking water.

Drink a minimum of half your body weight in ounces of water. If you weigh 160 pounds, you should drink 80 ounces of water or ten, 8 oz. glasses of water daily. If your urine is dark yellow or orange, that is a good indication that you are becoming dehydrated. Ideally, urine should be light yellow or colorless. Drink more than half your body weight of water if you feel you are dehydrated.

Tips for Drinking More Water

- When you first get up, drink at least two glasses of room temperature filtered water. This will help you relieve your bowels.

- Drink at least two more glasses before you leave home. Take glass-bottled water with you.

- Drink water while traveling to your destination.

- Upon arriving at your destination, drink water. By now you'll probably have to use the bathroom as well.

- If you work in an office, every time the phone rings, drink or sip some water.

- At lunch, drink 8 ounces of water before eating.

- Drink two 8 ounce glasses of water 2 hours after eating. Sip water instead of guzzling it down.

- When you arrive home in the evening, drink one 8 ounce glass of water.

- Whenever you feel hungry, drink water first. Many of us eat when we are really thirsty.

This should give you a minimum of eight glasses of water a day. If you need to drink less, make the necessary adjustments. Strive to drink enough water daily. Make it a conscious effort until it becomes effortless.

Drink water at room temperature. Water that is too cold or too hot causes the body to use more energy to absorb and process it.

Squeeze half a lemon into a glass of water. The combination of lemon and water eases heartburn and bloating, dissolves mucous, cleanses the liver and kidneys, and stimulates digestion.

Salt is an important nutrient in the body and goes hand-in-hand with water. When water and salt are combined, a third dimension is created that produces a higher energy form—sole, meaning "liquid light energy." Biologically when water and salt are combined, they give the body and mind everything it needs. Adding natural salt to water balances the

Good Nutrition

body's energy deficit and neutralizes the negative harmful electromagnetic vibrations in our body.

Dr. F. Batmanghelidj, author of *Your Body's Many Cries for Water*, recommends adding half a teaspoon of unrefined Celtic sea salt to the diet per day for every 10 glasses of water you drink.

Another option is to make a sole by adding the Original Himalayan Salt Crystals to water, allowing the water to become saturated to the point where no more crystals can be dissolved. At this point, undissolved salt crystals remain in the water. Add 1 teaspoon of sole to an 8 oz. glass of living spring water. Drink daily.

According to studies conducted by Peter Ferreira, co-author of *Water & Salt the Essence of Life*, drinking sole water daily can restore the body's natural frequency patterns, balance acid-alkaline imbalances, normalize blood pressure, dissolve metals, weaken addictions and heal skin diseases.

Factors That Influence Water Needs

- **Exercise** - The more you sweat, the more your water intake will need to be replenished. Hydrate before, during and after exercising. **Coconut water** from young Thai coconuts is naturally sweet, and a good source of electrolytes making it an excellent beverage to drink before and after exercising.

- **Environment** - Hot and humid weather and high altitudes require additional water intake. Heated indoor air can cause your skin to lose moisture in the wintertime.

Health Journey

- **Illness/Health Conditions** - Fever, vomiting and diarrhea cause the body to lose fluid. Bladder infections and urinary tract stones require increased water intake.

- **Pregnancy or breast-feeding** - The Institute of Medicine recommends that pregnant women drink 2.4 liters (about 20 cups) of fluids daily and that women who breast feed consume 3.0 liters (about 21.5 cups) of fluids a day.

Healing Waters

Biophysically water has the ability to carry information and energy through its crystalline cluster formation. To prove this, pioneer Japanese scientist, Dr. Masaru Emoto, developed a technique to photograph newly formed crystals of water samples. Dr. Emoto experimented by taking tap water and infusing it with negative spoken words and freezing it and photographing its image. Then he defrosted the SAME water and infused it with positive spoken words such as "I love you," froze it and photographed it. In each photo, the water appears to "change its expression." Go to www.hado.net to view these amazing photos of water crystal images.

Clearly water has great healing energy. Since ancient times, people have indulged the five senses in the healing powers of water. We indulge in ocean waters, therapeutic baths, hydrotherapy, hot springs, waterfalls, and holy springs. Why not use the spiritual power of prayer to ignite the healing powers in water? Let us infuse our water with love and gratitude by blessing our drinking water, singing while bathing and showering, and meditating while enjoying water sports.

WHOLE FOODS

Whole foods are taken directly from their sources and contain all of their original nutrients. Whole foods include fresh fruits, fresh vegetables, nuts, seeds, and whole grains.

Fresh fruits and vegetables contain a properly balanced amount of oxygen, water, enzymes, proteins, carbohydrates, vitamins, minerals, and phytonutrients.

Whole grains are the seeds of various types of plants including wheat, oats, barley, rye, millet, buckwheat, amaranth, quinoa (keen-wah), corn and rice. A grain is considered **whole** if all **three** of its layers are intact:

The bran: the outer layer, which is a rich source of B vitamins, phytonutrients, and 50-80% of the grain's minerals, and the majority of the grain's fiber.

The endosperm: the main part, which contains most of the grain's protein and carbohydrates and small amounts of vitamins and minerals.

The germ: the small inner core, which furnishes high amounts of B vitamins, vitamin E, some protein, trace minerals, healthful unsaturated fats, antioxidants and phytonutrients.

Scientific evidence demonstrates that eating a diet rich in whole grains has many health benefits:

- keeps the heart healthy and reduces risk of heart disease

Health Journey

- reduces the risk of certain types of cancers (colon, stomach)

- helps manage diabetes

- promotes regularity and maintains digestive health

- aids in weight loss

Whole grains can be found in cereal, bread, crackers, English muffins, granola, pasta, popcorn, rice, tortilla chips, etc. Look for the whole grain stamp to be certain you are getting products made with whole grains.

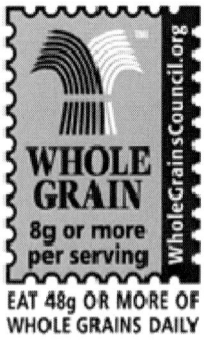
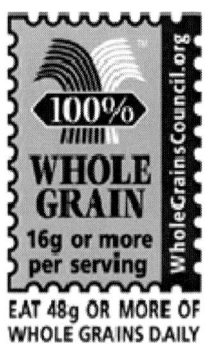

Whole Grain Stamp
For products offering a half serving or more of whole grain. Contains at least 8g whole grain per serving.

100% Whole Grain Stamp
For products where ALL of the grain is whole grain. Contains at least 16 g whole grain per serving.

Labels such as "bran", "multi-grain", "100% wheat", "cracked wheat", and "stone ground" **do not mean** products are made with whole grains.

Good Nutrition

Many excellent whole grain foods do not have the Whole Grain Stamp. Read the ingredients listed on the package for whole grains.

US Dietary Guidelines recommend that everyone eat 3 servings of whole grains daily. The USDA defines a whole grain serving as any food containing 16 grams, or half an ounce, of whole grain. Three servings (48 grams) of whole grain total less than two ounces.

Whole Grain Flour is milled from all three parts of the grain. It contains all the nutrients found in the seed (bran, germ, endosperm). Food made from this flour would be whole grain. Look for brands that are milled at low temperatures such as stone ground.

Refined Flour (all-purpose flour) has had the bran and germ and all of its nutrients stripped away.

If you avoid whole grains because you are intolerant to gluten, the following grains are gluten free:

- Amaranth - high in protein, lysine, and fiber. Good source of calcium, iron, potassium, phosphorus, and vitamins A, C, and E.

- Buckwheat - contains all 8 essential amino acids, vitamins B1 and B2, potassium, magnesium, phosphate and iron.

- Corn – high in thiamine, vitamin B5, folate, vitamin C, phosphorus, manganese and fiber.

Health Journey

- Flax - excellent source of omega-3 fatty acids, B vitamins, magnesium, manganese and phytonutrients.

- Millet - a good source of protein, fiber, niacin, thiamine, riboflavin, methionine, lecithin, vitamin E, iron, magnesium, phosphorous and potassium.

- Quinoa - contains all the essential amino acids, also high in iron, potassium, riboflavin, vitamin B6, niacin, thiamine, magnesium, zinc, copper, manganese and folic acid.

- Wild rice - high in protein, potassium, phosphorus, B vitamins.

Grains are very nourishing when grown, stored, milled, processed and prepared in the proper manner. Unfortunately, modern farming and processing practices have lead to overdependence on chemicals and hormone-like substances used in cultivating and storing grains.

Collection bins are sprayed with insecticide to "protect" against insects. Damp grains are dried artificially at high temperatures that denature the proteins and compromise its nutritional value. The high-speed mills produce high temperatures and high pressures that further destroy nutrients.

Store-bought bread, cereal, pasta, and rice have added preservatives and synthetic vitamins to replace those destroyed by refinement and milling.

Good Nutrition

Stored grains .will ferment within 90 days. This fermentation process creates fungus and mold. Mold produces poisonous chemicals known as mycotoxins. Mycotoxins increase acidity in the body, lower the immune system, raise LDL cholesterol, cause inflammation, allergies, eczema, candida, fatigue, depression, anxiety, PMS, ovarian cysts and infertility.

Spelt, amaranth, quinoa, millet, buckwheat, and wild rice are not stored. Sprout these grains to boost nutrition, assimilation and digestibility. Add food grade hydrogen peroxide, lemon juice, or ¼ teaspoon of vitamin C to soak water to reduce toxins.

Sprouting grains increases their vitamins, minerals, enzymes and nutrients such as proteins producing essential amino acids after germination. Sprouting also destroys phytic and oxalic acids found in grains and breaks down the gluten. Sprouted grains are loaded with fiber making digestion and elimination effortless.

Make your own flour, cereals and bread using sprouted grains. To make flour, once grains are sprouted, dry them using a food dehydrator at a low temperature. Grind the grains using a grain mill, coffee grinder or Vita-mix blender. To make cereal or bread, grind the sprouted grains using a food processor, Champion juicer, wheatgrass juicer or meat grinder.

Store dry seeds in a glass jar with a lid to keep moisture out. Canning jars are excellent for this purpose. Dry seeds will keep several months, but avoid storing them for more than three months.

Once the seeds are sprouted, store the sprouts in the refrigerator in a plastic or glass food container with a lid. Most sprouts will keep up to one week.

Health Journey

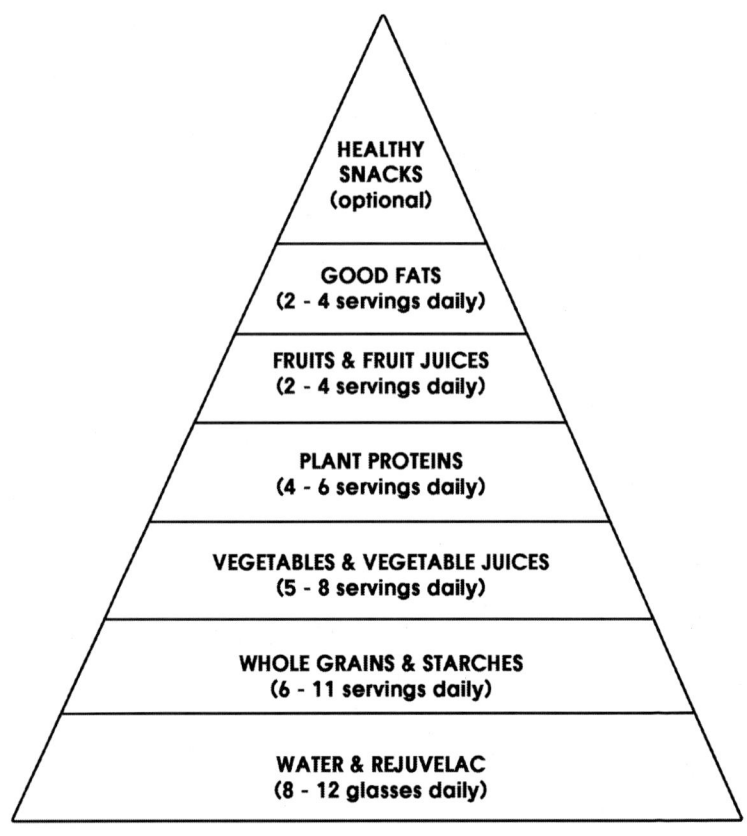

Plant-Based Food Guide Pyramid

Personalize your pyramid based on your caloric intake, weight, exercise level, metabolic rate and age. For example, if you are a very active young man with a high metabolic rate, you want to consume a higher amount of servings in each category. Pregnant and breast feeding women need more nutrients as well.

Rejuvelac is a fermented beverage made from sprouted grains and water. It gives you energy, aids digestion and elimination, and removes toxins from the body. For more information visit pages 88 and 108.

Good Nutrition

Recommendations for Better Health

We all have unique individual needs that require different amounts and types of foods to achieve optimal nutritional balance and performance. No one diet is right for everyone. You must be the one to determine the right foods in the right amounts for you.

Factors such as age, appetite, physical activity, emotional state, season, climate, and time of day influence what and how much we eat. Some people feel better with and require a high level of carbohydrates. Others need more protein-rich foods, and still others function better with a balance of both. Follow the guidelines below to determine what foods keep you balanced.

1. Keep a food journal for 7 consecutive days that includes what you eat, what time you eat, and how you feel before and afterwards. Pay close attention to how you feel after eating carbohydrates, proteins, and fats to determine how your body metabolizes each of them. Record findings in your food journal. Eat the foods that make you feel good.

2. When planning meals, make sure you include a balanced amount of each food group—carbohydrates, proteins, fats.

3. Plan food shopping in advance. Make a shopping list that includes a variety of fruits, vegetables, seeds, nuts and whole grains.

4. Drink at least eight, 8-ounce glasses of water daily.

5. Use the pyramid on the previous page as a guide to building a healthy foundation.

Health Journey

6. Eat a variety of fruits, vegetables, whole grains, nuts and seeds daily to ensure you are getting an abundance of nutrients

7. Avoid cooked starches such as rice, cereals, bread and pasta as they are difficult to digest and raise blood sugar levels.

8. Sprout grains such as quinoa, millet and buckwheat and make them your grains of choice.

9. Combine iron-rich foods with foods high in Vitamin C and foods that increase hydrochloric acid such as orange, lemon and lime juices.

10. Combine leafy greens in salads, juices and smoothies to form complete proteins.

11. Add sprouts to salads and blended soups to balance nutrition.

12. Replace saturated fats such as butter, margarines, lard and partially hydrogenated shortenings with nuts and seeds, and nut and seed oils.

13. Make sure you get a good amount of fiber found in plant foods for good elimination.

14. Flavor foods with fresh herbs and spices instead of table salt and irradiated seasonings.

2

FOODS TO AVOID FOR OPTIMUM HEALTH

PROCESSED FOODS

Processed foods are foods that have been stripped of their natural nutrients. Many processed foods contain artificial colors, flavors, hydrogenated oils, preservatives such as sodium (salt) and sugar, and toxic chemicals such as alloxan which is added to wheat when making white flour.

Processed foods include white flour and foods made with it such as pancakes, cakes, bread, bagels and pasta, pearled barley, white rice, table salt, white sugar, sweeteners, hot dogs, and most packaged snack foods.

Additives are put in food to extend the shelf life of processed foods, enhance flavor or color, improve nutritional value, and maintain food consistency.

Processed foods marketed as meat substitutes are made primarily from wheat gluten and soy protein isolate. Gluten is a mucous-forming toxin linked to digestive and respiratory disorders, diabetes, and hives. Refer to page 55 for more information on soy.

Refined Sugars

White sugar, brown sugar, high fructose corn syrup, molasses, and all of its derivatives are drugs. Natural

Health Journey

sugars are balanced by its nutritional makeup—vitamins, minerals, enzymes and fiber. Once the nutrition is isolated from the plant it becomes a drug.

The consumption of refined sugars robs your body of precious minerals and vitamins causing nutritional deficiencies. Nutrient deficiencies increase your appetite and cause you to eat more. Sugar is a simple carbohydrate that the body converts to sucrose. The liver then converts it to glucose for fuel. Any excess is stored in the liver as glycogen. When the liver's storage capacity is full, glucose is then converted and stored as fat.

According to the USDA, Americans consume an average of 152 pounds of sugars (caloric sweeteners) per person, per year. That's an average of 6 cups per week and 42.5 teaspoons per day. This is three times the amount of dietary sugars that is recommended.

In addition to sugar found in desserts, candy, crackers, bread and cereals, sugar is used as a preservative in processed foods, and can be found in canned foods, ketchup, peanut butter, mouthwash, toothpaste, even baby food. Fat-free and low-fat foods have high amounts of sugar added for flavor.

Consumption of sugars causes tooth decay, a suppressed immune system, Candida albicans (yeast overgrowth), enlarged liver and kidneys, hypertension, memory lapses, mood swings, and Diabetes II.

Soft drinks contain a whopping 12 to 15 teaspoons of sugar, carbon dioxide and phosphoric acid. Sugar robs the body of minerals and rots your teeth. Carbon dioxide robs the body of oxygen. Phosphoric acid dissolves bones and causes hardened arteries and joint disease. Aluminum cans leach aluminum into soft drinks, which can cause brain deterioration.

Bottled juices are loaded with preservatives. How is it that fresh juice that oxidizes quickly can be put in a bottle, and stored and still be fresh?   You are drinking rancid juice that looks and tastes good because chemicals have been added.

Artificial Sweeteners

As bad as refined sugar is, artificial sweeteners are worse. Just think toxic chemicals. Dangerous acid-forming chemicals have no place in your body!

Salt and Sodium

White table salt is a drug, because like white sugar, it has been isolated from its original natural source (salt crystals), and concentrated. Refined table salt is made of 66.66% elemental chloride and 34.34% sodium, as well as additives such as aluminum compounds to prevent caking and clumping. Much of the salt today is produced by trapping seawater and evaporating the brine and concentrating the salt by boiling it. This concentrating process removes the minerals and rearranges salt's molecular structure. Salt and sodium are used as flavor enhancers and preservatives for foods such as canned soups, cured meats, infant formulas, and cheese.   Excess salt and sodium consumption causes elevated levels of blood pressure (hypertension), and increases the risk of heart attack and stroke, dehydration, fluid retention, and accelerates aging. Natural sodium is found in grains, fruits and vegetables.

ANIMAL-BASED FOODS

Beef, pork, and poultry that you find in grocery stores and restaurants come from factory farms where they are fed genetically-modified grains laced with pesticides, herbicides, animal feces, and flesh from diseased animals. These animals are injected with high doses of antibiotics to keep them alive, and growth hormones and steroids to make them grow faster. The natural diet for cows is grass. Chickens are kept in overcrowded cages most of their lives.

Red meat is difficult to digest, and produces an excessive amount of uric acid. Uric acid is excreted through the kidneys. Too much uric acid in the urine places a dangerous burden on the kidneys, resulting in kidney stones. When the kidneys are overloaded, the muscles absorb and retain uric acid resulting in the formation of tiny sharp crystals causing rheumatism and neuritis (kidney inflammation). When these uric acid crystals are formed in the joints it causes gout, an extremely painful joint inflammation.

When you eat animal flesh, you are ingesting everything the animal has been fed, leading to serious health problems such as obesity, diabetes, infertility, kidney disease, precocious puberty and cancer.

Fish

Lakes, rivers, and oceans have become polluted with PCBs and mercury. Fish literally breathe the water they swim in, continually accumulating more and more toxins.

Though all fish are at the top of the food chain, tuna, bass, halibut, swordfish, and marlin show the highest

Foods to Avoid for Optimum Health

concentrations of mercury. Drugs are often administered in fish farming to control diseases that result from crowding.

Shellfish - there are two types of shellfish: mollusks (clams, oysters, scallops, snails, mussels) and crustaceans (shrimp, lobster, crab). Their feeding habits and their preference for coastal waters make them more likely to be polluted with toxins and pesticides.

Additionally, fish and shellfish are exposed to poisons from chemicals in the ice they are packed in for shipping.

Mercury and PCBs are both known toxins to humans that damage the nervous system, kidneys, liver and other organs, cause developmental disorders in children and pose a great health risk in pregnant women and their babies, and have been linked to cancer.

If you must eat flesh, wild Pacific salmon, Tilapia, Croaker, Sardines, Haddock, and Summer Flounder are the safest fish.

Dairy

Dairy products (milk, eggs, cheese, yogurt) found in grocery stores come from cows and chickens raised in dairy farms where they are subjected to similar treatment as animals raised in factory farms. Dairy products contain large amounts of cholesterol and saturated fats, a major cause of heart disease. Dairy products contain lactose, a milk sugar that most people are unable to digest and is often found to be the cause of digestive problems. The milk protein, Casein, has been shown to cause iron-deficiency anemia from internal bleeding in many infants and is suspected of causing juvenile diabetes.

Pasteurization takes the good things out with the bad. It kills beneficial enzymes, destroys colloidal minerals, destroys beneficial bacteria and lactic acids, destroys vitamins, and promotes other pathogens. Pasteurized milk and milk products contribute to allergies, osteoporosis, arthritis, heart disease, cancer, tooth decay, colic, disorders of the female reproductive system, and weakened immune system.

Nut and seed milks are a tasty and nutritious alternative to cow's milk. You can also make cheese and yogurt using nuts and seeds. (See recipes section).

COOKED FOODS

Cooking alters the molecular structure and nutrients of food. Depending on the cooking method, nutrients such as vitamins, minerals, and amino acids are depleted. Proteins are altered creating cross-links, which accelerate aging and bring about disease. Fats become rancid and cannot be emulsified. The water content is decreased. Enzymes are destroyed. Various carcinogenic and mutagenic substances are created, as well as many free radicals. All these factors make digestion, absorption and elimination of cooked foods incomplete which create a buildup of mucoid plaque in the intestines.

Eating cooked foods causes us to overeat because of the nutritional deficiencies. Our body is telling us it needs nutrients, so we keep eating. This cycle of overeating leads to overweight and obesity. When the

Foods to Avoid for Optimum Health

cells are not properly nourished and the body is overloaded with free radicals, toxins, and carcinogens, eventually it begins to break down and pre-mature aging and disease occur.

GENETICALLY MODIFIED ORGANISMS

Most of us have probably been exposed to genetically modified organisms (GMOs) without our knowledge or consent. Most of the foods in your local grocery store are now contaminated with GM food ingredients. The United States is one of the largest producers of GM crops. Soybeans and corn are the top two most widely grown crops. Other crops include tomatoes, cantaloupes, cotton, sugar beets, and Hawaiian pineapples. Sources of GMOs include meat, eggs, and dairy products from animals that have eaten GM feed, and dairy products from cows injected with the growth hormone rbGH. Highly processed foods, such as vegetable oils, breakfast cereal, corn meal, salad dressing, bread, margarine, mayonnaise, crackers, cookies, candy, chips, enriched flour, tomato sauce, and pasta contain some percentage of genetically-modified ingredients. Soybean derivatives in the form of food additives, meat substitutes, frozen yogurt, tofu, soy sauce, soy cheese, and soy protein powder are ubiquitous, ensuring that we all have been exposed to genetically modified food products.

Genetically modified foods are plants that have been modified in the laboratory to enhance desired traits such as herbicide tolerance, pesticide resistance, improved nutritional content, faster growth, and harder texture. Unlike conventional plant breeding methods, genetic engineering can create plants with the exact desired trait very rapidly and with great accuracy.

Health Journey

Excerpt from Seeds of Deception by Jeffrey Smith:

Health Risks

According to the Institute for Responsible Technology, there are about two dozen published, peer-reviewed animal feeding studies on the health effects of genetically modified foods.

- One study showed evidence of damage to the immune system and vital organs, and a potentially precancerous condition. When the scientist tried to alert the public about these alarming discoveries, he lost his job and was silenced with threats of a lawsuit.
- Two other studies also showed evidence of a potentially pre-cancerous condition. The other seven studies were not designed to identify these details.
- In an unpublished study, laboratory rats fed a GM crop developed stomach lesions and seven of the forty died within two weeks. The crop was approved without further tests.

The only human feeding trial ever conducted confirmed that genetically engineered genes from soy transferred to the bacteria inside the digestive tract. The biotech industry had previously said that such a transfer was impossible.

About 100 people died and 5-10,000 fell seriously ill when they consumed the food supplement L-tryptophan. Only those who consumed the variety that was genetically modified became ill. That brand had minute, but deadly contaminants that would easily pass through current regulations today. If the disease it

Foods to Avoid for Optimum Health

created had not been rare and acute, with crippling and deadly symptoms, the GM supplement might never have been traced as the cause. Once discovered, however, industry and government covered up facts and diverted the blame.

Milk from rbGH-treated cows contains an increased amount of the hormone IGF-1, which is one of the highest risk factors associated with breast and prostate cancer.

Soy allergies skyrocketed by 50% in the UK, coinciding with the introduction of GM soy imports from the US.

The Center for Disease Control and Prevention reports that food is responsible for twice the number of illnesses in the US compared to estimates just seven years earlier. This increase roughly corresponds to the period when Americans have been eating GM food. Could that be contributing to the 5,000 deaths, 325,000 hospitalizations, and 76 million illnesses related to food each year?

There are documented health risks of GM foods that warrant discussion and debate. These risks include evidence of reaction in animals and humans; gene insertion disrupts the DNA and can create unpredictable health problems; the protein produced by the inserted gene may create problems; the foreign protein may be different than what is intended; the transference of genes to gut bacteria, internal organs or viruses; GM crops may increase environmental toxins and bioaccumulate toxins in the food chain; other types of GM foods carry risks and risks are greater for children and newborns.

Health Journey

It is alarming that the biotech industry and the government are blinded by the myth that GM foods are needed to feed the world. It is even more alarming that they would gamble with our health and support their safety claims based on obsolete and unproven data.

The American public may likewise be foolhardy by accepting these assurances and eating these risky foods.

For more information, please read **Seeds of Deception**, by Jeffrey M. Smith, or visit the website at www.seedsofdeception.com.

CANOLA OIL

Canola is a hybridized, genetically engineered plant developed in Canada from the rapeseed plant, which is part of the mustard family of plants. Rapeseed oil contains a highly toxic substance known as erucic acid, and is poisonous to living things.

In the 1960s, scientists used plant breeding methods to get rid of erucic acid and glucosinolates, and canola was created. Although most of the erucic acid has been removed, canola oil still contains about 1% of this toxin. Today, 80% of the canola grown in Canada has been modified using biotechnology (GMOs) to make it tolerant to some herbicides to reduce the amount of chemicals needed for weed control.

Canola oil must be processed at high temperatures to remove the genetically-modified protein from the oil. This high heat processing transforms the polyunsaturated oils into toxic trans-fatty acids, and causes the omega-3s to become rancid and produce free radicals.

Foods to Avoid for Optimum Health

SOY PRODUCTS

According to extensive research conducted by the Weston A. Price Foundation®, soy phytoestrogens disrupt endocrine function and have the potential to cause infertility and to promote breast cancer in adult women.

Soy phytoestrogens are potent anti-thyroid agents that cause hypothyroidism and may cause thyroid cancer. In infants, consumption of soy formula has been linked to autoimmune thyroid disease.

Intake of phytoestrogens even at moderate levels during pregnancy can have adverse affects on the developing fetus and the timing of puberty later in life.

Babies fed soy-based formula have 13,000 to 22,000 times more estrogen compounds in their blood than babies fed milk-based formula. Infants exclusively fed soy formula receive the estrogenic equivalent of at least five birth control pills per day.

Premature development of girls has been linked to the use of soy formula and exposure to environmental estrogen-mimickers such as PCBs and DDE.

Megadoses of phytoestrogens in soy formula have been implicated in the delayed or retarded sexual development in boys.

High levels of phytic acid in soy reduce assimilation of calcium, magnesium, copper, iron and zinc. Phytic acid in soy is not neutralized by ordinary preparation methods such as soaking, sprouting and long, slow cooking.

Health Journey

Trypsin inhibitors in soy interfere with protein digestion and may cause pancreatic disorder. Only a long period of fermentation (two summers according to historical methods) will significantly reduce the phytate content of soybeans. Fermented soy products such as tempeh, miso, and soy sauce provide nourishment that is easily assimilated, but the nutritional value of tofu and bean curd, both high in phytates, is questionable.

Vitamin B12 analogs in soy are not absorbed and actually increase the body's requirement for B12.

Soy foods increase the body's requirement for Vitamin D. Toxic synthetic vitamin D2 is added to soy milk. Soy foods contain high levels of aluminum, which is toxic to the nervous system and the kidneys.

Soy beans are processed at very high temperatures to make soy protein isolate, and textured vegetable protein (TVP). As a result, the fragile proteins are denatured and toxic lysinoalanine and highly carcinogenic nitrosamines are formed. These soy products greatly inhibit zinc and iron absorption. Zinc is needed for optimal development and functioning of the brain and nervous system. Read more about iron on page 29.

Soy milk products and mock meats made with soy protein isolate and textured vegetable protein are used extensively in school lunch programs, commercial baked goods, diet beverages and fast food products.

For additional information about soy and references, visit www.westonaprice.org, and read *The Whole Soy Story* by Kaayla T. Daniel.

RECOMMENDATIONS FOR BETTER HEALTH

1. Pick a day to go through your kitchen and remove all canned foods, processed foods, packaged foods, foods made with hydrogenated oils, white flour, white rice, cake mixes, prepackaged pastries, fried chips, artificial sweeteners, flavors, and colorings, white sugar, gelatin and pudding mixes, ice cream, frozen yogurt, frozen microwaveable meals, sodas and juice drinks, whole-milk products, bottled salad dressing, mayonnaise, ketchup, peanut butter, vegetable oils, and processed meats (lunch meats containing carcinogenic nitrates).

2. Make a plan to eliminate meat, fish, dairy, fried foods, unfermented soy, ice cream, pizza, soda, caffeine, white sugar, table salt, and all junk and fast food from your diet completely. Start eliminating one thing at a time; i.e., one month all processed foods, the next dairy products, etc. Give your body a chance to adjust to the changes.

3. Eliminate all sugar substitutes such as Nutrasweet, Equal, Splenda, and Sweet & Low.

4. Add organic seasonal fresh fruits, vegetables (including sea vegetables), fermented foods, and sprouted whole grains to your diet.

5. Use only organic coconut and walnut oils; flax, olive, grape, hemp, pumpkin and sesame seed oils.

6. Never heat nut and seed oils, as they become rancid. Use coconut oil for cooking.

7. Replace white table salt with Celtic sea salt, celery powder, kelp or dulse flakes (sea vegetables).

Health Journey

8. Replace white refined sugar with stevia or agave. See pantry on page 94 for description.

9. Read package labels. If the food contains chemicals, preservatives, soy protein isolate, genetically modified organisms, or if you cannot determine what's in it, don't buy it.

10. Avoid soy milk, ice cream, cheese, mock meats and other packaged foods containing wheat gluten and soy protein isolate such as seitan, soy bacon, ham, sausage, hot dogs, hamburgers and waffles.

11. Decrease the amount of cooked foods and increase the amount of raw foods eaten at meals.

12. Join in the campaign to inform society of the truth about soy.

13. Stay abreast of legislature concerning GMOs and push for GMO labeling of foods.

14. Attend PTA meetings and get involved with food advocacy.

15. Share what you know with others by screening films and holding lectures in your home or at school. For more information, check out these websites:

   Informedeating.org
   Thechinastudy.com
   Foodpolitics.org
   Prwatch.org
   Naturalovens.com
   Thefutureoffood.com
   Truecostoffood.org
   Foodstudiesinstitute.org

3

GOING GREEN!

The planet is suffering from the effects of greenhouse gases, holes in the ozone, air pollution and acid rain, water pollution, modern living, chemical toxins, and too much waste. It is our responsibility to make it better.

THE GREENHOUSE EFFECT

Greenhouse gases produced by carbon dioxide (CO_2), nitrogen oxide, and methane pollute the atmosphere and cause the atmosphere to heat up. Carbon dioxide is produced by the burning of fossil fuels such as coal, oil, gasoline; and wood. Nitrogen oxide is given off when we drive our vehicles and by power plants that burn coal to generate electricity. Methane is created by rotting plants and by household garbage. Even when we pass gas, methane is created!

The Greenhouse Effect upsets the balance of nature causing the oceans to warm up, as well as higher sea levels, flooding, and warmer temperatures.

Sea water and sea organisms called plankton soak up CO_2 in cold water. Plants and trees, particularly those in the rainforest, help soak up CO_2. But as the oceans heat up, the water is not cold enough to soak up CO_2. Trees in the rainforests are being cut down and burned to create farmland for raising beef. As a result, there are fewer trees to soak up greenhouse gases, and the burning of trees produces even more CO_2 contributing to the greenhouse problem.

Health Journey

HOLES IN THE OZONE LAYER

There are many large holes in the ozone layer. One is the size of the United States and growing. These holes are caused by a family of chemicals called chlorofluorocarbons (CFCs) used in manufacturing hundreds of products that we use everyday including bicycle seats, furniture cushions, cameras, computers, TVs, radios, jewelry, plastics and foam packaging such as egg cartons. When these chemicals are released into the atmosphere and interact with sunlight they release chlorine atoms that attack and destroy parts of the ozone layer.

AIR POLLUTION AND ACID RAIN

Air pollution affects humans, animals, plants, trees, crops and forests. Pollution from power plants, cars, buses, mowing the lawn and even barbecuing exposes us to toxic chemicals that pollute the air and cause many illnesses.

Acid rain poisons fish, kills trees, damages buildings and causes disease and health problems in humans, particularly babies, seniors, and people with asthma and bronchitis. Acid rain is created when sulfuric acid mixes with moisture. Sulfuric acid is formed when sulfur dioxide or nitrogen oxides are mixed with water. Sulfur dioxide and nitrogen oxides are primarily caused by the burning of coal that contains high levels of sulfur and the burning of fossil fuels, including gasoline burned in automobile engines and oil used for cooking and heating.

WATER POLLUTION

The pollution of our water supply by the farming industry and industrial waste has put our lakes and rivers at risk of drying up. This puts our lives at risk because we cannot survive without clean water.

CHEMICAL TOXINS

Plastic water and baby bottles, and food and beverage can linings such as those used for baby formula, contain a chemical called bisphenol A (BPA) that can leach into food and beverages. Plastic manufacturers maintain that the levels that leach into food are well below the safety thresholds set by the Environmental Protection Agency (EPA).

But many scientists disagree, stating that the industry-funded studies were flawed, and that new independent studies reveal the potential for harm. In 2007, the Environmental Working Group (EWG) reported that BPA posed an urgent health threat to infants on canned formula because infants eat so much more than adults per pound of body weight. The EWG's report linked BPA to increased cancer-cell growth, gene activity, and hormonal development of infants. Visit www.ewg.org for more information.

Again the American public finds itself in the middle of a controversy over the safety of chemicals and practices that affect our health. In these situations I think it best to exercise caution to preserve our good health.

Environmental chemicals are not only found in our food supply, but also in cosmetics and cleaning products. Antibacterial soaps, body washes, fragrances, toothpaste, towels, plastic cosmetic containers, nonstick cookware, stain-resistant clothing, microwave popcorn bags, and drinking water all contain toxic chemicals that affect our health.

MODERN LIVING

Modern living has placed us in disharmony with nature. Somewhere along the way we have lost respect for the Earth and its many inhabitants. Thousands of plants, animals, and insects that humans need for survival are destroyed when the rainforests are cut down, and as many as 6,000 species are forever lost every year because of logging. Many animals have become endangered so that we can wear fur, ivory, corals, leather, and use beauty creams.

TOO MUCH TRASH

Modern living has created a throwaway nation. As we consume more and more, we waste more and more. Every time you buy something, you immediately throw away the package it came in. Think of all the things you buy—food, electronics, cosmetics, appliances, furniture. These items create a lot of trash. Where does that trash go? Eighty percent ends up in landfills or dumps. Ten percent is recycled and the other ten percent is incinerated. Much of what we throw out is not biodegradable, creating a need for land to fill with our garbage. What will we do when we run out of landfill space? Where will we put all our garbage?

And how should we dispose of the products such as batteries, plastics, inks used on packages, and disposable diapers that contain hazardous substances that can seep into the ground and contaminate the air, water, and soil?

GOING GREEN GUIDELINES
How Can We Live in Harmony With Nature?

- **Reduce energy usage!** Walk, bike, take the bus, train or carpool to work. Turn off the lights when leaving a room. Prepare raw foods and use your stove less. Get your head out of the refrigerator and close the door! Replace light bulbs with long-lasting, low-energy bulbs.

- Set your thermostat a few degrees lower in the winter and a few degrees higher in the summer.

- Get a water filter and install a low-flow shower filter. Plastic bottles are not biodegradable and fill up our landfills. If you must drink bottled water, use a Nalgene #2 high density polyethylene bottle.

- Bring your own bag to the grocery store to avoid plastic and paper bags.

- Cut down on packaging by buying products with little or no packaging as much as possible.

- Avoid fast food. Not only is it unhealthy, but most is packaged in styrofoam that cannot be recycled.

- Cut your water usage in half. Only flush when you need to. Take shorter showers and only run the dishwasher when it is full.

- Recycle as much as you can. Set up recycling bins for paper, glass and aluminum. Look for the recycling symbol on toilet paper, tissues, computer paper, and food packages. Use cloth napkins, dishtowels and sponges instead of paper towels.

Health Journey

- Reuse and buy used. Use rechargeable batteries. Shop at thrift stores for household items and clothes, or trade clothes with someone your size.

- Compost your food scraps. Use it for fertilizer.

- Properly dispose of hazardous waste such as batteries, old paint, used motor oil, unused pesticides and weed killers. Call your local city office for hazardous waste disposal guidelines.

- Use non-toxic cleaning products. Make your own with vinegar, fruit and baking soda.

- Purchase natural soaps, toothpaste and cosmetics made with organic ingredients. Avoid using aerosols. They cannot be recycled.

- Buy or can your own fruits and vegetables in safe glass jars. Choose canned foods from makers who don't use BPA, such as Eden Foods.

- Use glass baby bottles or plastic bag inserts made of polyethyelene, or switch to reusable polypropylene bottles that are labeled #5.

- Go vegetarian! Industrial meat production requires too much energy and creates harmful waste that is damaging to the environment, and to our health.

- Visit these websites for more information: www.thegreenguide.com, www.worldwatch.org, www.ivillage.com, www.sierraclub.org.

Support sustainable practices. Sustainable farmers work with nature to produce more wholesome food while using less fossil fuel (thus lessening the impact on global warming), and without using any synthetic pesticides, artificial hormones, or antibiotics.

Sustainable farmers do not take more resources to produce food than they give back. Thus, sustainable food production can be maintained indefinitely. Reliance on renewable resources, as well as on symbiotic relationships with nature and the surrounding community, means that these farms do not damage the environment, are humane to workers and animals, provide fair wages to the farmers, and support and enhance rural life.

Buy and eat locally grown food. Food from local sustainable farmers tastes better, is fresher, and is more nutritious. It is better for the environment and cheaper. Food that has traveled hundreds of miles must be picked before it is ripe, stored and transported, adding to fuel costs, and global warming. Purchasing from local farmers helps to keep them in business and protects farmland from becoming developed. Most important, buying locally supports the local economy.

Eat foods in season. Support sustainable practices by buying and eating fruits and vegetables that are in season where you live. Such produce will be fresh and abundant in vitamins and minerals.

Health Journey

Buy Organically Grown Produce

Organically grown produce is grown without pesticides, herbicides, fungicides or chemical fertilizers. By choosing organic, you are minimizing exposure to the 8,000 chemicals used in conventional farming. Here are 8 good reasons to buy organic fruits, vegetables, nuts and seeds:

1. Organic foods taste better and are higher in nutrients.

2. Certified organic products carry a guarantee. Certification is the public's guarantee that products have been grown and handled according to strict procedures without toxic chemical inputs.

3. Organic production reduces health risks by reducing the number of exposures to toxic chemicals.

4. Organic farmers build soil. Soil is the foundation of the food chain and the primary focus of organic farming. By building healthy soil, plants are better able to resist disease and insects.

5. Organic farms respect our water resources. Each small piece of living soil contains thousands of microorganisms that help retain water and provide nutrients to the plants. Consequently, organic agriculture requires less water.

6. Organic producers lead in innovative research aimed at reducing pesticides and minimizing agriculture's impact on the environment. Production techniques include cover cropping, use of beneficial insects, crop rotation and diversification, botanical and biological pest control, composting, close

Going Green

observation of natural soil, plant and wildlife systems, and cultural mechanical weed control.

7. Organic farming helps keep rural communities healthy. Organic farming is one of the few survival tactics left for the family farm and the rural community.

8. Organic farmers work in harmony with nature. Organic agriculture represents the balance demanded of a healthy ecosystem; birds and insects control pests; wild life is an essential part of a farm and is encouraged by including forage crops in rotation and by retaining fence rows and wetlands.

If you cannot eat all organic foods, beware of these 12 foods that contain the most contaminants: strawberries, green and red bell peppers, spinach. US cherries, peaches, cantaloupes, celery, apples, apricots, green beans, grapes, and cucumbers

When eating conventional produce, rinse in a solution of 1 ounce of 35% food-grade hydrogen peroxide (sold in health food stores) to 1 gallon of water. The oxygen neutralizes toxins on the surface of the produce.

Peel all waxed produce before eating including squash, bell peppers, eggplant, cucumbers, tomatoes, potatoes, apples and papaya.

Health Journey

RECOMMENDATIONS FOR BETTER HEALTH

1. Implement the going green guidelines immediately. Share these guidelines with everyone you know.

2. Implement a recycling program at work if one does not already exist.

3. Find out what's in season where you live. Only buy what's in season.

4. Shop at a farmer's market, or join a CSA (community supported agriculture) group or a food co-operative. They are better sources for obtaining local, seasonal produce at affordable prices.

5. Support fair trade products that ensure that farmers get a fair price for their commodities.

6. Ask your local supermarket, schools and hospitals to carry organic foods.

7. Shop at local businesses that support sustainable and responsible business practices.

8. Eat organic produce whenever possible.

9. When eating out, select restaurants that use organic ingredients. Be mindful of foods prepared with heated oils.

10. Don't be fooled by packaged foods that are advertised as natural and organic. Once all the nutrients are processed out of the food and preservatives are added, the benefits are destroyed.

4

CULTIVATING GOOD HABITS

EAT JUST ENOUGH

Why do we eat so much? Is it because we love to eat so much that we can't stop until we have eaten everything? Is it because our parents made us clean our plates when we were young before we could leave the table? Is it because what we are eating does not have enough nutrients and our bodies are starved? Is it because we are feeding our emotions by eating to feel better?

Many factors influence how much we eat. Sometimes it has to do with what we are doing while we are eating, the size of the dish or package we are eating from, the way the food is plated, and who we are eating with.

Whatever the cause, overeating is a bad habit that must be broken. Overeating even healthy foods can be detrimental to one's health. The damage is cumulative, but each day the body degenerates a little more. Overeating can lead to food addictions, destructive behavior, illness, indigestion, constipation, obesity, rheumatism, diabetes II and premature aging.

We tend to overeat starchy foods, particularly when emotionally stressed. These foods cause a slow rise in blood sugar and make us feel good which causes us to eat too much. Additionally, starchy foods are usually loaded with salt and sugar.

Health Journey

If you think overeating is not a problem, check out these statistics:

- 66% of Americans are overweight
- 31% of Americans are obese
- Childhood obesity in the US has more than tripled in the past two decades
- 60% of African American men in the US are overweight
- 78% of African American women in the US are overweight
- 29% of African American men in the US are obese
- 51% of African American women in the US are obese
- 300,000 deaths each year in the US are associated with obesity
- Overweight and obesity are associated with an increased risk of heart disease, certain cancers such as colon, gall bladder, prostate, kidney, and postmenopausal breast cancer, type 2 diabetes, stroke, arthritis, breathing problems, and psychological disorders, such as depression
- A weight gain of 11 to 18 pounds increases a person's risk of developing type 2 diabetes to twice that of individuals who have not gained weight

The problem is that we have no idea of how much we are eating. When dining out, as the majority of us do, the portion sizes in restaurants are huge, and we usually feel obliged to get our money's worth by eating everything on our plate. Add to this appetizers and dessert; we leave feeling stuffed and ready for bed.

Cultivating Good Habits

Here are a few suggestions to help gain control over how much you eat.

1. Cut your portions in half. Only put half of what you think you are going to eat on your plate. If you desire more after eating, wait 10 minutes before eating more.

2. Use a smaller plate, and it will look full.

3. When eating out alone, order an appetizer as your main course instead of an entrée.

4. When eating out with others, share an entrée.

5. Do not overeat. Stop eating when you first feel full.

6. Eat only when hungry.

7. Drink water at the first sign of hunger.

8. Chew your food well. Practice chewing your food at least 20 times before swallowing. Chewing your food ignites the digestive enzymes and begins the process of digestion. Chew your food well for good digestion, assimilation and elimination.

9. Eat slowly, taking small bites and putting down utensils between each bite.

10. Never eat out of a bag or carton. Portion out food in a container prior to eating and put the rest away.

11. Eat three moderate meals a day.

12. Avoid snacking between meals.

Health Journey

13. Limit the number of items eaten at a meal. See the food combining chart on the following page for clarification.

14. When choosing to eat the foods you like that you know are unhealthy, eat half the amount you normally would. Eat less and less of those foods until you no longer desire them.

15. Be conscious of serving sizes. Check the serving size listed on the Nutritional Facts panel on food labels. All of the nutrients (carbohydrates, proteins, fats, sodium, etc.) listed on the food label are based on the serving size. If you eat more than one serving, the amount of nutrients, as well as calories and fat, will increase.

WHAT CONSTITUTES A SERVING?
Use dry measuring cups to measure ingredients

- ½ cup fresh fruit, veggies, pasta, meat, fish
- 1 slice of bread
- ½ hamburger bun, or ½ English muffin
- 3 ounces of meat, poultry (size of computer mouse)
- A small handful of nuts
- ½ cup cooked cereal, rice or pasta
- 1 ounce ready-to-eat cereal
- A medium apple, banana, or orange
- A grapefruit half
- A melon wedge
- ½ cup berries
- ½ cup cooked vegetables
- ½ cup chopped raw vegetables
- 1 cup leafy raw vegetables
- ¼ cup cooked rolled oats

PROPER FOOD COMBINING

Good health cannot be realized in an acidic body. Contributing factors include eating acid-forming foods and combining foods that require different digestive environments (acid or alkaline) in the body to be digested well. The effects of poor food combining are cumulative. Each day there is a little fermentation with absorption of the products, and each day the body degenerates a little until one day the body can no longer continue.

Proper food combining will help you maintain an alkaline digestive tract, which will enable you to digest food well, absorb its nutrients, and eliminate waste efficiently, and consequently avoid illness and disease that thrives in an acidic digestive environment.

Bloating, burping, constipation, fatigue after eating, upset stomach, gas and heartburn are results of poor food combining.

When eating living foods, combining principles are much more relaxed because difficult to digest foods such as beans, nuts, and seeds are soaked and sprouted to increase alkalinity and digestibility. In effect they are "pre-digested," meaning that through the sprouting process, the nutrition is broken down into usable units such as amino acids, simple sugars and fatty acids. Consequently, when eating living foods, you have more flexibility and can combine foods that would not be recommended if cooked.

The following are guidelines for proper food combining. Remember we are all unique, and they may not all apply to everyone.

Health Journey

FOOD COMBINING GUIDELINES

Liquids Alone. Drink liquids *(water, lemonade, grass juice, fruit and vegetable juices, coffee, tea)* before your meal and wait 15 minutes before eating, or drink liquids after what you have eaten has left the stomach. Drinking liquids with the meal dilutes the hydrochloric acid in the stomach, making digestion less efficient. Liquids carry food out of the stomach before they are completely broken down.

Do Not Combine Dense Proteins *(meat, fish, eggs, dairy)* **with Dense Starches** *(bread, cereal, corn, crackers, grains, potatoes, pasta, yams)*. Proteins are digested in an acid medium in the stomach. Starchy carbohydrates are digested in an alkaline medium in the mouth.

Fruits Alone. Fruits digest quickly, and should be eaten alone to avoid fermentation.

Do Not Combine Acid Fruits *(Lemons, Limes, Pineapples, Kiwi)* **with Sweet Fruits** *(Bananas, Dates, Figs, Prunes, Raisins)*. Acid fruits require a more alkaline digestive environment than sweet fruits.

Melons Alone. Melons contain more water than other fruits and require less time in the stomach.

Watermelon Alone. Watermelon consists of mostly water and its required time in the stomach is less than that of other melons.

Cultivating Good Habits

LENGTH OF TIME FOODS STAY IN THE STOMACH

Water	10-15 Minutes
Juice	15-30 Minutes
Rejuvelac	20-30 Minutes
Nut Milk	30-45 Minutes
Fruit	30-60 Minutes
Melons	30 Minutes
Watermelon	15 Minutes
Sprouts	60 Minutes
Wheat Grass Juice	60-90 Minutes
Barley Grass Juice	60-90 Minutes
Most Vegetables	1-2 Hours
Grains and Beans	2-3 Hours
Sprouted beans, seeds, legumes	1-2 Hours
Soaked Nuts	1-2 Hours
Dense Vegetable Protein	2-3 Hours
Cooked Meat and Fish	3-4 Hours
Shellfish	8 hours

Try eating non-starchy vegetables like **broccoli, cauliflower, and zucchini** with dense protein and starch. So instead of eating meat with potatoes, eat meat with vegetables, and potatoes with vegetables.

Sub-Acid fruits **(apples, berries, apricots, cherries, mangoes, papayas, peaches, pears and plums)** can be combined with sweet fruits **(dates, raisins, figs, bananas)** or acid fruits **(oranges, pineapples, pomegranates, sour grapes, grapefruits, lemons)**.

It is best to sprout beans, seeds, and legumes. Once sprouted, they are vegetables for the purpose of food combining.

Health Journey

ALKALINE-FORMING FOODS

Fresh Fruits - All fresh fruits and fruit juices are alkaline-forming except for blueberries, cranberries, plums and prunes.*

Fresh Vegetables - All vegetables* are alkaline-forming.*

Grains - Amaranth, millet and quinoa are alkaline-forming grains.* Acid-forming grains such as barley, buckwheat, rye, spelt and wheat become alkaline-forming when sprouted. Sprouting alkaline grains make them even more alkaline.

Beans - Fresh green, lima and string beans are alkaline-forming as well as fresh green peas and snap peas.* As with grains, acid-forming beans such as Adzuki, black, chickpeas, kidney, lentil, mung, navy, pinto, red and white beans become alkaline-forming when sprouted. Beans form complete proteins when combined with grains.

Nuts - Aside from almonds and fresh coconuts, nuts are slightly acid-forming. Soaking nuts make them alkaline-forming.*

Seeds - All sprouted seeds are alkaline-forming.*

Herbal Teas - All alkaline-forming.

*Cooking, freezing, canning, pickling and preserving with sugars and chemicals greatly reduce alkalinity.

Meat, refined and cooked salt, sugar and starches, alcohol, coffee and soft drinks are acid-forming.

JUICING

Juicing fruits and vegetables is a delicious way to get the daily vitamins, minerals, enzymes, purified water, proteins, carbohydrates and chlorophyll we need. Instead of taking supplements, I prefer to juice. Because the fiber is separated from the juice, your body receives the nutrients from the juice in a concentrated, balanced form.

Juicing allows you to eat more fruits and vegetables than you would normally eat, in combinations that you would never consider. Particularly when drinking green vegetable juices, you can combine many leafy greens and herbs such as kale, arugula, dandelion, celery, parsley, and watercress to make a tasty beverage. However, it is unlikely that you would combine these vegetables if you were going to eat them. So juicing also allows you to ingest a variety of fruits, vegetables and herbs.

Worldwide, people have found healing from ailments such as chronic fatigue syndrome, high blood pressure, heart disease, arthritis, anxiety, depression, sleep disorders, and many other conditions through juicing. In addition to fresh wheat or barley grass, I drink a fresh fruit or green juice daily.

Fruit juices cleanse and energize the body. Select fruits in the acid and sub-acid categories to avoid consuming too much concentrated sugar.

Green vegetable juices build and regenerate the body. For optimum digestion, combine green vegetable juices with carrot, celery, lemon, lime or water in a 2:1 ratio.

Health Journey

JUICING GUIDELINES

1. Begin with fresh organic produce.

2. Wash produce with a biodegradable vegetable wash or a solution of food-grade hydrogen peroxide.

3. Juice citrus fruits--oranges, limes, tangerines and grapefruits in a citrus juicer.

4. Remove pits and large seeds from fruits such as plums, cherries, peaches, and apricots.

5. Cut produce to fit your juicer's feed tube.

6. Use stems and leaves of most produce, except carrots.

7. Strain juice after juicing to remove additional pulp.

8. Only make what you will drink right away. Drink immediately as fresh juice oxidizes quickly.

9. If you must store juice, do so by placing a thermos in the freezer over night. In the morning prepare the juice. Pour it in the thermos letting it spill over to prevent any air space. Screw the top on tightly. When drinking the juice from the thermos, drink all of it at once. Do not drink some and recap it.

10. Avocadoes, mangoes, bananas, papayas and melons do not juice well. Blend them with fresh juices to make soups, puddings and smoothies.

11. Once the juice turns brown it has oxidized. Do not drink it.

JUICE FASTING

Juice fasting is simply drinking fruit and vegetable juices, and pure water, instead of eating. Because you are getting your nutrients in a liquid form, they will enter the bloodstream much quicker and allow better absorption of nutrients.

Juice fasting can be a very effective way to control diet, eliminate illness and disease and increase one's life span. Let's face it we eat too much of the wrong foods, have too much stress in our lives, do not exercise enough, don't get enough sleep, and sometimes drink, drug and party. It's just a matter of time before these things catch up with us. When they do, it's time to fast!

Fast when you don't feel like yourself, when you are stressed, when you are constipated, when you have diarrhea, when you have indigestion, when you have a headache, when you have a stomach ache, when you can't sleep, and when you are sick and tired. These are signs of toxicity. Help the body out by fasting to cleanse and heal the body.

Fasting relaxes the body and begins the healing process. It allows the digestive organs to rest, cleanses the liver, kidneys, tissues and colon, and purifies the blood. Your eyes will be clear and bright, your breath will be fresh, you will be slimmer, you will sleep like a baby and awaken fully refreshed and ready to go, and most importantly, you will experience a peacefulness that will lead you to self discovery.

I recommend fasting with the seasons for a minimum of three days. The first two days are the hardest (at least for me). On the third day the healing begins. If a three day fast is a breeze for you, try fasting for longer the next time. Fast until you feel the urge to eat again. Begin and break a fast by eating blended foods for half the length of the fast. Break the fast with fresh applesauce. It is imperative to take enemas or have colonics while fasting.

> *"To lengthen thy life, lessen thy meals"*
> **Benjamin Franklin**

Juice fasting is an excellent way to practice calorie restriction. One factor in human longevity researchers agree on is a low-calorie diet. Specifically: **a diet high in good nutrition and low in calories**. Since 1935, numerous studies have suggested that caloric restriction is the only strategy to date that has been scientifically proven to extend the maximum life span.

Researchers suggest that if you want to live substantially longer, you must reduce your caloric intake by 10, 20 or even 30 percent. Diseases such as heart disease, stroke, cancer, diabetes, osteoporosis and Alzheimer's can be avoided or forestalled.

Benefits of a Calorie Reduction Diet

- Helps reduce free radicals
- Delays age-related immunological decline
- Helps to lower insulin levels and improve glucose-insulin metabolism
- Increases the body's ability to repair damaged DNA, thereby renewing cells
- Slows metabolism, making it more efficient
- Reduces the age-related decline in melatonin levels

COLON CARE

Good elimination is essential to good health. Most of us suffer from some form of constipation. Even eating a predominantly healthy diet, one can get backed up because there are many factors that influence good elimination. Let's take a look:

- Drinking enough water to hydrate the colon and stimulate peristalsis. Dehydration is a major cause of constipation;

- Having a balance of soluble and insoluble fiber, such as flax meal in the diet;

- Having enough lubrication (healthy fat) for smooth and gentle elimination;

- Getting enough exercise to stimulate the lymphatic flow to create peristalsis;

- Taking medications including anti-depressants, pain relievers, antacids, diuretics, antibiotics, and even supplements that contain binders;

- Not having enough time to eliminate completely causes constipation. The more relaxed you are, the better the elimination; and

- Traveling disrupts your normal routine. Many people are often constipated when traveling.

When we are eliminating properly, we should have 2 to 3 bowel movements a day—in the morning when we get up, after lunch, and after dinner.

Health Journey

What happens when you eat 3 or more times a day and do not eliminate 3 times a day? Where does the waste go?

The large intestine (colon) is 5 feet long and 2-3 inches wide and can store encrusted mucous mixed with fecal matter called mucoid plaque for decades! It is believed that the average person stores up to 25 pounds of waste accumulated over the years in their colon, stretching the colon walls up to 5 times its original size—hence an expanded midsection.

This waste causes toxins to enter the bloodstream through the intestinal wall, which can lead to malabsorption and self-poisoning called autointoxication.

Once toxins settle into the tissues, it can cause headaches, brain fog, depression, obesity, diverticulitis, PMS, bad breath, indigestion, gas, bloating, arthritis, body odor, and more serious disorders such as colon cancer.

Certainly drinking more water, increasing bulk and lubrication will increase elimination, but what about the damage that has already been done? What about all of the waste that has accumulated in your body for years? How do we bring the colon back to health?

Enemas! There are two types of enemas: cleansing and retention. The cleansing enemas are used to flush out the descending colon removing fecal matter from the colon walls, and releasing incomplete bowel movements that have hardened. To begin you will need an enema bag. Fill the bag with warm water (around 101°F). Use a thermometer to test the water. Add 2 ounces of fresh wheat or barley grass juice to

Cultivating Good Habits

purify the water. You can also use coffee and Rejuvelac instead of water in your enemas to stimulate peristalsis and pull toxins from the colon.

After the cleansing enema, a Retention enema (also called implants) can be taken to help replenish electrolytes lost during the cleansing enema. An implant is done by putting 4 ounces fresh wheat or barley grass juice in your enema bag and holding it up to 10 minutes before releasing. In the beginning it will not be possible to hold the implant for 10 minutes. Always release when you feel the need to. Eventually you will be able to hold it for 10 minutes. Fresh grass juices are easily absorbed into the bloodstream when used as an implant, detoxify the colon and liver, and help cleanse and rebuild the colon by destroying putrefaction bacteria. Taking an enema and implant 2 to 3 times per week will help to bring the colon back to health and reduce the effects of toxicity.

If enemas are not for you, consider getting a **colonic**. A colonic uses more water and cleans the entire colon-- descending, transverse and ascending colon. Colonics are administered by a hydrotherapist. Fecal matter leaves the body through a tube.

Once toxins are leached into the blood stream, the liver, kidneys, lungs, lymphatic system and skin are affected as well as the colon. Herbs can be effective in facilitating elimination, cleansing the organs and detoxifying the body. Purgative herbs like cascara sagrada, senna and pharamaceutical laxatives are habit forming and impair the colon's ability to function on its own. Gentle minerals and herbs like magnesium hydroxide, aloe and rhubarb bring water into the colon instead of purging it out, and stimulate peristalsis.

Health Journey

RECOMMENDATIONS FOR BETTER HEALTH

1. Work up to eating 80% alkaline and 20% acid foods.//
2. Thoroughly chew your food, even blended foods.
3. Stop eating two hours before going to bed.
4. Never eat when upset or angry.
5. Try not to overeat. Practice portion control. Stop eating when you first feel full.
6. Practice the food combining principles, particularly when eating cooked food.
7. Have a least one fresh juice daily.
8. Take digestive enzymes with meals, particularly when eating cooked food.
9. Allow enough time to go to the bathroom in the morning. This may mean getting up earlier.
10. Position yourself correctly when using the toilet. Keep the feet raised on a telephone book or stool.
11. Take enemas regularly (2-3 times per week), or get a colonic once or twice a month.
12. Fast with the seasons or when you feel the need to. Always take enemas daily when fasting!
13. Find an herbalist to prescribe herbs to cleanse all the digestive organs.

5

ADOPTING A PLANT-BASED DIET

By now it is obvious that a plant-based diet offers the most nutrition for good health. For me personally, becoming vegetarian was a turning point in my life. I used to be a very angry and aggressive young woman who would get up in your face and tell you off at the drop of a hat and slam the door behind me. But when I became vegetarian, all of that anger subsided, suggesting that it wasn't me who was angry, but the animal I was ingesting. I felt peaceful inside. Let me tell you, when you are at peace with yourself, it is very difficult to be mean and rude to others. In addition to losing weight, my health improved and I experienced true happiness for the first time in my life. But it wasn't until I became vegan that I experienced optimum health.

Vegans do not eat eggs or dairy products like vegetarians, and they rely exclusively on plant foods to meet their nutritional needs. Further, vegans abstain from participating in an industry that sacrifices animals for the sake of beauty, fashion and furniture.

Most people are vegetarians for health reasons. Vegetarians tend to be leaner and have a lower incidence of hypertension, coronary artery disease, colon and lung cancer, type II diabetes, and diverticulitis.

The production of meat, dairy, fish and poultry degrades our land, wastes water, and pollutes the rivers and streams at the expense of mankind.

Ethically we know it is wrong to harm animals. Hopefully one day meat eaters and vegetarians will come to respect all life forms, and abstain from eating meat, dairy, fish and poultry through the realization that a plant-based diet is the best diet for healthy people, healthy animals and a healthy planet.

RAW AND LIVING FOODS: FOR OPTIMUM NUTRITION, FLAVOR AND DIGESTIBIITY!

Once you have purchased fresh organic food, you want to ensure that the flavor and nutrition are not cooked away. Remember that up to 90% of vitamins and minerals and all enzymes contained in foods are destroyed when heated above 118°F.

The best way to get all of the nutrients and flavors of whole foods is to prepare them at low temperatures, or eat them raw.

Raw Foods are foods prepared without cooking, but they are sometimes sprouted, marinated, fermented, and blended to make them more digestible, and dehydrated (below 118°F) to add variety.

When raw food is sprouted and fermented, it is considered a **living food**. There are many active enzymes, vitamins, minerals, antioxidants, and phytonutrients in raw and living foods.

People are generally surprised at how good raw food tastes. Spices are intended to enhance the flavor of food, but when they are heated, the spices become overpowering, and flavor of the actual food is masked.

Adopting A Plant-Based Diet

Even when eating a raw salad, most of us put so much dressing on it, we cannot taste the vegetables.

Raw and living foods are so delicious because you can taste all of the flavors of the ingredients in the food. Your taste buds will sing with joy. And because the enzymes are not cooked away, you feel energized after eating raw foods instead of feeling tired. Enzymes are protein molecules that are essential to every function of life. Digestive enzymes break down carbohydrates, proteins, and fats into usable units such as simple sugars, amino acids and fatty acids, making digestion much more efficient and effortless.

Blending foods makes them easy to digest. It helps us to chew our food (which most of us do not do well). Remember when you were a baby, you ate blended foods? Blended foods are so easy to make and are delicious and nutritious. They include smoothies, soups, sauces, dips, dressings, and puddings. You will need a heavy duty blender, but always start with what you have and go from there.

Marinating. Raw leafy greens and vegetables can be very difficult to digest. To make them more digestible, we marinate them by adding oil and salt, and using the fire from our fingers to massage them and break them down. Marinating increases digestibility, and adds variety to a raw foods diet.

Dehydrating. Dehydrated foods are foods that you would normally bake, but instead you dehydrate them at a low temperature to keep the enzymes, vitamins and minerals intact. Dehydration provides us with some of the textures of cooked food, and the taste and nutrition of raw food. Dehydrated foods add variety and help us overcome addictions to unhealthy snacks.

We use a food dehydrator to make cookies, crackers, loaves, burgers, breads, pizza crusts, spices, fruit leathers, and to warm food.

Fermenting. Early civilizations used fermentation as a way of preserving foods, and making toxic foods edible. Fermentation introduces friendly *lactobacilli* to your digestive tract to break down food, assimilate nutrients and create B vitamins (folic acid, riboflavin, niacin, thiamin, and biotin), omega-3 fatty acids and many other nutrients.

Live food cultures such as sauerkraut, kim chee, miso and soy sauce, and beverages such as kombucha and Rejuvelac promote healthy friendly bacteria and can help control diarrhea, dysentery and bacteria such as E-coli and Salmonella. Many people take pro-biotics to increase friendly bacteria, but many are pasteurized and do not contain live cultures. Fermenting live foods yourself is much more cost effective and beneficial.

What's Rejuvelac? Rejuvelac is a fermented beverage made by sprouting wheat berries or any grain, and letting them soak in water for several days. After 3 days, the water is strained, and you have Rejuvelac!

Rejuvelac was created by Ann Wigmore, the founder of the Ann Wigmore Institute. Rejuvelac aids digestion and elimination due to the fermentation process. It contains a very high level of enzymes that replace enzymes that cooked foods have depleted. When made with wheat, it contains vitamins A, B, E and K. It also has the friendly bacteria necessary for a healthy colon which helps to remove toxins from the body. See recipe section to make Rejuvelac!

Grass Juices

Grains such as wheat, barley, rye and oats produce a grass when planted. Once they are harvested, the grass can be juiced and drunk. Grass juices contain 70% chlorophyll which is essential in protecting, healing and repairing the human body. Chlorophyll detoxifies and rebuilds the blood stream, improves circulation, cleanses the organs and gastrointestinal tract, heals gum disease and ulcers, creates an unfavorable environment for bacteria, neutralizes the polluting elements in food, air and water, and low-level radiation, freshens the breath and neutralizes body odors, improves blood sugar and improves skin problems such as acne, eczema and psoriases. Grass juices help restore a high energy level by fulfilling nutritional deficiencies and removing toxic wastes that clog our cells, blood, tissues and organs. They increase stamina, aid digestion and elimination, reduce cravings for addictive substances, improve fertility, inhibit the growth of disease-causing bacteria, and the activity of cancer-causing chemicals.

When grown in organic soil, grass absorbs 92 of the known 102 minerals from the soil, and contains all eight essential amino acids. The two most popular grasses are barley and wheat.

Barley Grass Juice is high in chlorophyll, flavonoids, beta carotene, enzymes, all the essential amino acids, calcium, iron, magnesium, phosphorus, copper, manganese, zinc, vitamins B1, B2, B6, B12, C, E, folic acid, and pantothenic acid.

Wheat Grass Juice is high in vitamins A, B, E and K, and contains calcium, phosphorus, sodium, potassium, magnesium, iron and zinc.

Health Journey

I recommend drinking one to two ounces of wheat grass or barley grass juice a day. Consider it your multivitamin!

Algaes

Algaes are a group of one-celled plants, containing no true root, stem or leaf. They are found in freshwater ponds and lakes. This ancient superfood is the most nutrient dense food on the planet, containing chlorophyll, vitamins, including B12, minerals, complete proteins, simple carbohydrates, enzymes, and fats.

Chlorella is a whole green algae known for its high chlorophyll content, CGF (Chlorella Growth Factor) which allows it to multiply in less than 24 hours, and its natural balance of insoluble and soluble fibers and iron that cleanse the intestinal tract and bloodstream.

Spirulina is a blue-green algae that thrives in very warm waters, making it one of the cleanest foods found in nature. It is very easy to digest due to its soft cell wall, and contains a perfect balance of essential amino acids, vitamin B12, and beta carotene.

Blue-green algae grown wild in Upper Klamath Lake, Oregon, contain the highest amount of chlorophyll and vitamin B12, as well as a full spectrum of vitamins, minerals, complete proteins, carbohydrates and fats.

All of these products are grown, harvested, dried and packed using technology to protect and preserve its biologically active vital nutrients.

Adopting A Plant-Based Diet

Nuts

When transitioning to a live food diet, nuts are used to add nutrition, flavor and variety. Nuts are a good source of protein, fiber, phytonutrients, antioxidants, plant sterols and healthy poly and mono unsaturated fats. When eaten in moderation as part of a varied diet, nuts can lower LDL cholesterol and reduce the risk of heart disease and diabetes II.

A skilled chef will use different types of nuts to achieve desired flavors and textures in creating dishes that we are familiar with. Let's take a look.

Almonds – up until quite recently, almonds were the nut of choice because of their sweet delicate flavor and high calcium and vitamin E content. However, as of September 1, 2007, the Almond Board of California and the USDA created a mandatory program requiring that all raw almonds be pasteurized. This means raw almonds grown in the United States are no longer available for purchase from a retailer. Even if they are labeled raw they are not!

Brazil nuts are a good source of the antioxidant selenium, calcium and magnesium, and have a nice savory flavor. They are good in making burgers and nut meats, and add crunch to crackers and chips.

Cashews have a creamy texture and are used to make ice cream, creams, sauces, and pie and cake fillings. Cashews are an excellent source of iron, magnesium, phosphorous, potassium and zinc. Cashews are encased in a toxic liquid to which heat is applied to dry and remove the cashew, and consequently are not raw.

Health Journey

Hazelnuts (Filberts) have a sweet nutty flavor and are quite crunchy as well. They are mostly used in making milk and desserts. They are high in iron, magnesium phosphorus, potassium, thiamin and niacin.

Hemp nuts are easily digestible and the only complete source of protein, essential amino acids and essential fatty acids. They are high in calcium, magnesium, phosphorus, potassium and vitamins A, B, C, D and E. Hemp nuts are used to make nut meats and granola, and are sprinkled over salads or used in a crust.

Macadamia nuts are a good substitute for almonds and cashews. They have a slightly sweet, creamy, rich flavor and make a great pâté, milk, dessert filling, pie crust, sauce, cream and "cheese". Macadamia nuts have the highest fat and calorie content of any nut, and are high in magnesium, copper, thiamin, and iron.

Peanuts are not nuts they are legumes. They are contaminated with aflatoxin, a harmful fungus and they must be heated to remove toxins. Peanuts should not be used in raw food preparation.

Pecans have a buttery flavor, and are excellent in dessert crusts or savory dishes such as pâtés, nut meats, and stuffing. They are high in phosphorus, thiamin, copper, zinc, iron and potassium.

Pine nuts are tiny nuts with a nice buttery flavor. They are used to make salad dressings and sauces, and are sprinkled on salads. They are a rich source of potassium, manganese, magnesium, copper and zinc.

Walnuts are excellent in savory dishes such as burgers, pâtés, "cheese", pie crusts, and just about anything! They are a good source of omega 3 fats, phosphorus, zinc, copper, thiamin, iron and potassium.

Sprouted Seeds

Pumpkin seed sprouts from hulled pumpkin seeds are high in omega 3 fats, zinc, protein, and fiber. They have a distinctive taste and add flavor to pâtés, soups, nut meats and casseroles or are great as a snack.

Sesame seed sprouts from hulled sesame seeds are very small, and loaded with flavor. Use sprouted sesame seeds to make tahini, baba ganoush, falafel, milk, bread, Gomashio, salad dressings and nut meats. They are high in calcium, iron, magnesium, potassium, zinc, thiamin, riboflavin, and phosphorous,

Sunflower seed sprouts from hulled sunflower seeds are a rich source of folic acid, magnesium, niacin, phosphorous, potassium and zinc. They are a staple in thickening soups, making nut meats, pâtés, salads, crusts and desserts.

Storage

Buy fresh raw nuts and seeds from a busy health food store that stocks them in bulk bins and replenishes stock frequently.

Nuts and seeds contain mono and poly unsaturated fats, and will go rancid if not stored properly. They should be placed in an air-tight container and stored in a dark, cool, dry place like your refrigerator or freezer. Raw nuts and seeds will keep 2 months .in the refrigerator and 6-12 months in the freezer.

Health Journey

PANTRY

Make these items your staples. Use them in place of oils, salt, vinegar, and flavorings you've gotten rid of. They can be purchased at health food stores.

Agave Nectar (uh-gah-vay) — is a natural fructose from the agave plant, and is a healthy alternative to white sugar, honey, corn syrup and artificial sweeteners.

Apple Cider Vinegar — made from fermented apple cider. It is very high in minerals and promotes healthy digestion. Purchase organic, raw, unfiltered apple cider vinegar.

Celtic Sea Salt — salt from seawater harvested in Britanny. It is slowly dried in the sun to preserve marine micro-organisms, enzymes and some 70 other minerals and trace minerals. Celtic sea salt helps digest carbohydrates, proteins and fats, and increase stomach acid.

Coconut Oil — its very rich and buttery consistency is lower in fat than most fats and oils. Its naturally saturated fat content makes it ideal for cooking.

Flax Seed Meal — is high in protein including all the essential amino acids, Omega-3 oil and fiber.

Miso — a fermented bean paste of many varieties, both sweet and salty. Look for unpasteurized miso as it is a living food containing natural digestive enzymes, lactobacillus, and other micro organisms.

Nama Shoyu — an organic, live, unpasteurized soy sauce aged several months to several years. It is rich in enzymes and *lactobacillus* for a healthy flora balance.

Nutritional Yeast — a yellow, flaky yeast generally grown on molasses. It is not a raw product, but it has a wonderfully "cheesy" flavor and is abundant in many nutrients, including vitamin B12.

Sea Vegetables — are an excellent source of minerals, high-quality protein, enzymes, vitamins, and antioxidants. They have an alkalizing effect and help detoxify the body. Sea vegetables include arame, dulse, hijiki, kelp, kombu, wakame, and Irish moss.

Olive Oil — is produced from the fruit of the olive tree. It is considered cold-pressed if you purchase the extra virgin first pressing of the olive, which means it is unrefined and unheated.

Raw Carob Powder — used as an alternative to chocolate and cocoa, but it still contains caffeine and should be used sparingly.

Sesame Oil — is antibacterial, anti-inflammatory, antiviral, antioxidant and antifungal. Organic, cold pressed sesame oil has many healing and therapeutic qualities and can be used topically and internally.

Stevia — a sweetener extracted from the whole stevia leaf. It is sweeter than sugar and has a glycemic and caloric index of 0. It is also high in vitamins and minerals. Avoid white refined and alcohol extracted products. Stevia should be green like the leaf.

Vanilla Extract — a dark amber-brown liquid made from vanilla beans. Look for brands without alcohol.

SETTING UP A RAW KITCHEN

Get off to a good start by organizing your kitchen to make preparation as easy as possible. Having the proper tools and equipment is necessary to achieve desired results.

Chef's Knife

A good chef's knife is your most important tool in the kitchen. Purchase the best-quality knife you can afford. A high-carbon steel blade is recommended as it is the most durable material. Try it out in the store if possible, noticing how it feels in your hand. A good knife should have balance like an extension of your arm.

Cutting Boards

Cutting boards are essential. Quality wood cutting boards help extend the life of your knife by creating the least resistance against the edge of a knife. Avoid cutting on ceramic, metal or plastic surfaces which would quickly dull a knife's sharp edge, and are more likely to harbor bacteria.

Caring for Wooden Boards

After purchasing a wooden cutting board, rub on generous amounts of food grade mineral oil (warmed at room temperature) and allow oil to soak in. Repeat the process about 6-8 hours later and repeatedly if necessary until the oil is no longer being absorbed. Then wipe off any excess that remains on the surface.
Food grade mineral oil is tasteless and odorless. It does not get sticky and does not become rancid with time. It is available at supermarkets or drug stores.

Adopting A Plant-Based Diet

Wash your wooden utensils without worry after oiling. But **do not let wood utensils soak, and do not wash them in a dishwasher.** Wash your cutting boards after each use with warm soapy water, then rinse and towel dry. Wood dries faster than plastic, and will thus be less likely to harbor bacteria on its surface.

Bowls and Containers

You will need stainless steel bowls in a variety of sizes for soaking nuts, seeds and grains, and for mixing.

Glass or plastic food storage containers with lids are optimum for storing food. They will keep contents fresh longer than using plastic storage bags.

Where to Purchase Equipment

A restaurant supply store usually offers the most variety and best price for knives, cutting boards and bowls. A supermarket, drug store, or 99 Cents Store is ideal for purchasing food grade storage containers.

Sprouting Equipment

I like to use colanders for sprouting. Plastic or stainless steel can be used and purchased at a 99 Cents store or hardware store. Other sprouting equipment includes:

- Nylon Sprout Bags - good air circulation. Nice for traveling
- Hemp Sprout Bags - good for sprouting small seeds and grains.
- Glass jars - also good for small seeds, and for keeping bugs at bay

Storage Jars

Glass storage jars with lids are essential for storing nuts, seeds, and grains.

Food Processor

A high-quality food processor enables you to process vegetables, grains, and nuts to a variety of consistencies. Cuisinart is a time-honored favorite brand. Look for a 7 to 11 cup capacity. Most models have an "S" blade that lies low in the drum and is sharp enough to grind nuts, carrots and fibrous vegetables. Robo Coup is another good brand, though a bit pricier.

Blender

A high-speed blender is essential. Household blenders are unable to adequately process or achieve the desired smoothness when blending hard nuts and seeds. The motors will quickly burn out with this type of use. Recommendations:

- Vita Mix is the best of the blenders. It is expensive, but is well worth the money as it comes with a 7 year warranty.

Web sites that offer competitive prices and deals are:

- www.living-foods.com.
- www.vita-mix.com (includes 30-day guarantee). Or you may call Vita-Mix directly at 800-848-2649
- www.kitchen-universe.com
- www.instawares.com

Adopting A Plant-Based Diet

Juicer

There are so many juicers to choose from. Finding the right juicer for you will take some research. When selecting a juicer keep in mind the following:

- Is it easy to clean?
- How often will I use it?
- Will I use it for juicing or homogenizing?

For juicing fruits and vegetables I recommend the Breville Juice Fountain Elite. It retails for $300.00, and comes with a 1-year limited warranty. It has a stainless steel micro mesh filter and casing. The extra wide feed chute fits whole apples, carrots, tomatoes, and peeled oranges. It comes with a large pulp container, and a one liter juice jug. To purchase call 1-866-273-8455.

The Jack LaLanne is modeled after the Breville, but has less horsepower and plastic casing.

For juicing fruits, vegetables, grass and homogenizing, the Samson 6 in 1 GB-9001 is ideal. It retails for about $240. Call Samson directly at 888-992-7333 or visit the website at www.samsonjuicers.com. Juicersdirect.com is a good source for juicers.

Wheat Grass Juicer

A wheatgrass juicer is needed to juice grass. The electric model makes the job of juicing effortless, but the hand crank model will also extract the juice efficiently. The Healthy Juicer does a nice job, and juices other fruits and vegetables as well. Contact the manufacturer directly at www.healthjuicer.com. The Miracle electric wheat grass juicer is a good electric wheat grass juicer available at juicersdirect.com

Health Journey

Dehydrator

A food dehydrator with a thermostat adds new dimensions to raw food preparation. Excalibur is a good model. The heat is evenly distributed and controlled and it is not necessary to rotate shelves. Contact Excalibur directly at 800-875-4254 or www.excaliburdehydrator.com. The website www.livingright.com also has good deals. Their phone number is 800-432-2488.

Spiral Slicer (Spirooli)

A spiral slicer is used for creating angel hair, linguini or ribbon "noodles."

Measuring Devices

These include measuring spoons, liquid measuring cups, dry measuring cups, portion scoops (ice cream), and ladles. Using the proper measuring devices could mean the difference between success and failure.

When making a new recipe, follow the measurement guidelines given in the recipe using the proper equipment. Once you have become experienced at food preparation, you will get to know certain measurements and will be able to eyeball it.

Spatulas

Spatulas come in many different sizes and shapes. An offset spatula is great for spreading flax crackers, pizza crusts and breads to give them an even finish.

THE SIX TASTES

Combining the six basic tastes of sweet, sour, salty, pungent, bitter and astringent in dishes will ensure a balance of flavor and satisfaction.

Sweet tastes are calming, moistening and soothing and increase body bulk. Good choices include bread, sprouted grains, nuts, most fruits, starchy vegetables and oils. Spices: fennel seed, cinnamon, cardamom, poppy seed, anise, dill, tarragon, and nutmeg.

Sour tastes stimulate the appetite and digestion, increase metabolism, and help to dispel gas. Good choices include oranges, grapefruits, berries, fermented foods (sauerkraut), and tomatoes.

Salty tastes are warming, calming and drying. In small quantities they help to simulate appetite and digestion. Good sources are celery, Celtic sea salt, sea vegetables and olives.

Pungent tastes are commonly thought of as hot. They increase metabolism, circulation and digestion, and are helpful in lowering body fat, blood pressure and cholesterol. Good choices include chili peppers, garlic, onions, radishes, cayenne, cloves, ginger, cinnamon, cardamom, cumin, thyme, sage and turmeric.

Bitter tastes are dry and cooling. They aid in reducing body fat, and have disease fighting properties. Good choices are broccoli, cauliflower, kale, and cabbage.

Astringent tastes are drawing, drying, and cooling. They aid in the reduction of body fat. Good choices are beans, green apples, pears, green grapes, green tea, thyme, nutmeg, sage, and rosemary.

MEAL PLANNING

Eating a diet of raw and living foods does not have to be bland or boring. Choosing to eat healthy does not mean you must sacrifice taste for nutrition. You can have both. It is a good idea to start your transition to live foods by adding raw foods to what you are already eating. For instance, if your lunch consists of a sandwich and soup, make the soup a raw soup or have a salad instead. Add fresh sprouts to salads. Carry your own sprouts when eating out.

Start by planning meals ahead of time to allow enough time to soak and sprout. Never cut corners when it comes to sprouting. Plan meals for a week at a time and involve family members in planning and preparation.

It is wise to take time to plan meals on your day off. In the beginning keep it simple. Always keep in mind nutrition and food combining when planning meals. Select recipes that have similar ingredients. Raw food will last for several days.

Include snacks like nuts and seeds when planning meals. Make sure you have ample healthy snacks around the house, so when the urge hits you, you are prepared.

Experience has taught me that this path is not about being perfect. It's about trying your best each and every day, and being at peace with that. Some days are better than others. The perfection lies in the imperfection because that's where the lessons are. As they say in AA, stick with it--it works! I wish you love, happiness, joy and awesome health and vitality. You deserve it!

FOOD PREPARATION GUIDELINES

1. Always prepare food with spiritual consciousness. Think loving thoughts while preparing food. This alone will contribute to making great tasting food. Never prepare food while angry, depressed or sick. Food has energy and the energy you put into the food will be tasted, felt and absorbed. When we eat food prepared with love, we increase our love of God with every mouthful.

2. Use these recipes as a guideline. Always taste your dishes and adjust flavors according to your liking. Make dishes your own.

3. Incorporate the six tastes to ensure balance and satisfaction.

4. Be creative. Don't be afraid to experiment. Some of our best recipes have been so-called mistakes. Once you have become accustomed to adding raw foods to your diet, begin to experiment with recipes you already know how to make, but make them raw. That's how we began. We started with our favorite foods--collard and mustard greens. We discovered that re-creating these dishes raw was fun and, surprisingly, more tasty than the cooked version. From there we went to pizzas and burgers, which are now two of the most popular dishes on the menu at Raw Soul.

5. Preparing food for people is a big responsibility. Take it seriously. Take the time to hand chop vegetables whenever possible. Over processing food robs it of vital nutrients and life force.

Health Journey

6. Preparing live food is joyful! Approach it with enthusiasm and patience and you will succeed.

Good Hygiene

We all have harmful bacteria and viruses (germs) inside of us and on our bodies. The bacteria from our nose, throat, hair, skin, infected cuts, bruises and from our feces all cause food borne illnesses. We must be careful to prevent bacteria from getting into the food. When preparing food for other people, always practice good personal hygiene. Here are some suggestions:

1. Wear clean clothes, including a clean apron.

2. Avoid wearing jewelry, since it can collect dirt or fall off while working with food. Do not wear perfume.

3. Use a hat, cap, hairnet or other method to keep hair away from your face, hands and food.

4. Use a clean bandage and disposable gloves on a fresh uninfected wound.

5. Keep fingernails clean and trimmed.

6. Do not smoke, eat or drink while preparing food.

7. Wash your hands thoroughly and often:
   - Before starting to prepare food
   - Before putting on gloves
   - After using the toilet
   - After handling raw food
   - After touching your hair, or any part of the body
   - After sneezing or coughing
   - After handling non-food items

6

RECIPES

Soaking and Sprouting

Live food preparation begins with the soaking of nuts and sprouting beans, peas, grains and seeds. Soaking is the first step of sprouting. Soaking releases the enzyme inhibitors, acids and phytates making digestion of these foods effortless.

Always start with organic raw seeds. Begin by soaking in twice the amount of filtered water as seeds. Add liquid kelp, a solution of food-grade hydrogen peroxide or fresh squeezed lemon juice to soak water to help neutralize toxins and boost nutrition. Soak times will vary based on the size of various seeds. Use the chart on the following page as a guide.

Once nuts are soaked, rinse them well and strain them and they are ready for use. After soaking, beans, grains and seeds must be sprouted to make them more digestible, nutritious and flavorful. During germination carbohydrates, proteins and fats are broken down into usable units—simple sugars, amino acids and fatty acids thereby increasing digestibility. Sprouting is economical. You will end up with more than you started with (about two to three times as much). Keep this in mind when using recipes that call for sprouts.

You can use a kitchen colander, nylon sprout bags, hemp sprout bags, glass jars and baskets to sprout various foods. I like to use a kitchen colander because

Health Journey

it is easy and something that most of us already have. When sprouting beans and grains, a hemp sprout bag is preferable to avoid fungus and mold. The nylon sprout bag is great for travel. The basket is great for small vegetable seeds such as alfalfa, clover, fenugreek and radish.

Colander Sprouting Method

1. Strain soaked beans, seeds or grains into a colander and rinse.
2. Place the bowl underneath the colander to drain.
3. Put a dish towel over the colander and let sit in a well ventilated area. Do **not** put in the refrigerator.
4. Rinse before going to bed and cover again.
5. Rinse the next morning and cover.
6. Continue rinsing and covering twice a day until you see a small tail. This is the sprout.

Sprout Bag Sprouting Method

1. Place the soaked seeds in the sprout bag.
2. Hang the sprout bag on your towel rack to dry.
3. Rinse twice a day by immersing the bag in a bowl of cold water for 30 seconds or until the water is no longer cloudy.
4. Hang sprout bag to dry after each rinsing.
5. When you see a small tail your sprouts are ready.

Always use filtered water for soaking and rinsing.

Glass jars and baskets can be used for sprouting using the same principles as above, but must be inverted to allow for good drainage.

Recipes

Sprouting times will vary depending on temperature and humidity. Once you see the tails, they are ready. For best results, use sprouts immediately.

Seed	Amount	Soak Time	Sprout Time
Beans and peas	1 cup	8 hours	2-3 days
Amaranth	1 cup	4 hours	1-2 days
Barley (hulled)	1 cup	8 hours	2 days
Buckwheat	1 cup	6 hours	1 day
Kamut	1 cup	6 hours	2 days
Quinoa	1 cup	4 hours	½ day
Spelt	1 cup	6 hours	2 days
Wheat	1 cup	6 hours	1 day
Brazil nuts	1 cup	8 hours	
Cashews	1 cup	4 hours	
Flax seeds (whole)	1 cup	4 hours	
Hazelnuts	1 cup	8 hours	
Hemp Nuts/Seeds	1 cup	None	
Macadamia Nuts	½ cup	4 hours	
Pecans	1 cup	6 hours	
Pine Nuts	1 cup	None	
Walnuts	1 cup	6 hours	
Pumpkin Seeds	1 cup	6 hours	2-3 days
Sesame Seeds	1 cup	6 hours	1 day
Sea Vegetables	1 cup	½ hour	
Sun-dried Tomatoes	1 cup	2 hours	
Sunflower Seeds	1 cup	6 hours	1 day
Dried Dates & Raisins	1 cup	3 hours	

Oats, rice and millet have had their husk removed and will not sprout. To store sprouts, place them in a covered container and put in the refrigerator. They will keep for about 3 days or more depending on the type. Rinse well before using.

BEVERAGES

Rejuvelac (1 gallon)

1 cup sprouted wheat berries (or grain of choice)
1 gallon filtered water

Rinse sprouts thoroughly. Place sprouts into a blender. Add 1½ cups of water. Blend on high speed for 5 seconds. Pour into a gallon glass jar. Fill glass jar to the top with filtered water. Cover jar with a sprout bag or cheesecloth and secure with a rubber band.

Let sit at room temperature for 3 days until the taste is tart, like unsweetened lemonade. You will see a film at the top, this is *lactobacillus*. Strain the liquid into a gallon pitcher, using the sprout bag or cheesecloth. Discard seeds. Refrigerate. Drink Rejuvelac daily. It will keep in the refrigerator up to two weeks.

Variation

Add fruit, dates and raisins to the basic Rejuvelac recipe after placing the seeds in the glass jar and before filling it with water. Continue as above.

Mucous Eliminator (8 oz.)

1 grapefruit
1 orange
1 lime

Juice fruit using a citrus juicer. Strain and serve. Drink daily to eliminate mucous. Place peels in a gallon pitcher of filtered water. Use for drinking water

Yammy Pineapple Juice (8 oz.)

1 yam or sweet Potato
⅓ pineapple
1 pear

Wash and cut fruit. Juice, stir and serve.

Gratifying Green Juice (8 oz.)

For those of you who have difficulty drinking green juice, this is the perfect combination.

1 handful spinach or kale
1 handful dandelion greens
3 stalks celery
1 cucumber
2 limes
¼ inch fresh ginger (optional)

Wash ingredients. Juice all ingredients. Strain. Drink right away.

Bill's Real V8 (1 quart)

12 carrots
5 celery stalks
1 tomato
½ red bell pepper
½ cucumber
1 handful spinach
1 handful parsley
Pinch of ginger (optional)

Wash vegetables. Combine all ingredients in juicer. The ginger can easily overwhelm this drink, so use it sparingly. Strain, stir and serve.

Fruit Cocktail (16 oz.)

2 sweet apples
1 bunch red grapes
8 strawberries
¼ lemon

Wash fruit and juice. Serve.

Citrus Elixir (16 oz.)

5 oranges
1 grapefruit
1 lemon or lime
3 apples
5 strawberries
1 kiwi peeled
1 bunch grapes

Juice oranges, grapefruits and lemon or lime in citrus juicer. Juice remaining fruit in regular juicer. Combine both juices. Stir. Serve cold.

Sesame Milk (2 cups) *High in Calcium*

1 cup sesame seeds, soaked and strained
½ cup raisins, soaked with 4 cups filtered water
¼ teaspoon alcohol free vanilla extract

Blend all ingredients, including raisin soak water, until smooth. Strain through a cheesecloth. Serve chilled.

Coconut Milk (about 2 cups)
Meat and water from 1 young Thai coconut

In blender, blend all ingredients until creamy.

Recipes

Nut Milk (4 cups)

Brazil nuts, hazelnuts and macadamia nuts make healthy and delicious milks. Each offers its own unique flavor and nutritional makeup.

1 cup soaked nuts of choice
4 cups filtered water

Place nuts and water in blender. Blend until creamy. Strain through a cheesecloth to remove pulp. Add agave and/or vanilla extract if desired. Serve immediately or chilled. Use pulp to make cheese or cookies.

Strawberry Smoothie (1 serving)

1 cup nut milk of choice
1 cup fresh strawberries
1 tablespoon agave nectar

In blender, blend all ingredients until creamy. Serve.

Mango Lassi (2 servings)

Meat from 1 Young Thai Coconut
1 cup Rejuvelac
1 mango, peeled and cut
1 cup fresh orange juice
3 tablespoons fresh lime juice
Agave nectar to taste
¼ teaspoon ground cardamom seeds

In blender, blend all ingredients until creamy. How much agave you need will depend on the sweetness of the mango. Serve immediately or chilled.

SAUCES

Sauces are the key to adding flavor to a dish! Use over "pasta", "rice," vegetables, and nut meats to create fabulous dishes the entire family will love.

Mushroom Gravy (1 cup)

5 Shitake mushrooms, de-stemmed, chopped
1 chopped portabella mushroom
1/2 chopped onion
2 cloves chopped garlic
3 tablespoons nama shoyu
½ cup filtered water
1 tablespoon fresh tarragon, chopped
1 tablespoon fresh parsley, chopped

Place all ingredients in blender. Blend on high until very smooth and creamy. Add water if gravy is too thick. Pour in serving dish. Serve immediately.

Marinara Sauce (4 cups)

2 cups soaked sun-dried tomatoes
2 cups fresh chopped tomatoes
1 cup fresh chopped basil
2 cloves garlic
2 tablespoons lemon juice
6 pitted dates
2 tablespoons olive oil
1 teaspoon Celtic sea salt or nama shoyu
1 cup filtered water

Combine all ingredients in blender. Blend until smooth, adding water as needed.

Pesto Sauce (4 cups)

2 cups pine nuts
2 cups fresh basil
2 cups fresh parsley
¼ cup lemon juice
2 cloves garlic
Celtic sea salt to taste
2 cups filtered water

Blend all together in Vita Mix or blender.

Sweet and Sour Sauce (2 cups)

3 cups soaked sun-dried tomatoes
1 cup chopped red bell pepper
½-inch piece fresh ginger, peeled
1 clove garlic
2 tablespoons agave
1 tablespoon apple cider vinegar
1 tablespoon olive oil
1 teaspoon Celtic sea salt
1 cup filtered water

Combine all ingredients in blender. Blend until smooth.

Chili Sauce (2 cups)

3 cups soaked sun-dried tomatoes
1 small chipotle pepper, chopped
1 tablespoon chili powder
1 tablespoon cumin powder
1 teaspoon garlic powder
1 teaspoon Celtic sea salt
2 teaspoons agave
1 cup coconut water

Combine all ingredients in blender. Blend until smooth.

NUT AND SEED CHEESE

Remember fermented foods are abundant in enzymes, B vitamins, and good bacteria for good digestion!

Walnut Cheese

3 cups soaked walnuts
¼ cup lemon juice
1 tablespoon white miso
3 tablespoons nutritional yeast
½ teaspoon Celtic sea salt
Water as needed

In a food processor blend all ingredients to a smooth texture, adding water as needed.

Seed Cheese (2 cups)

⅔ cup soaked hulled sunflower seeds
⅓ cup soaked unhulled sesame seeds
3 cups Rejuvelac

Strain and rinse sunflower seeds in very warm water to remove skins. Strain and rinse sesame seeds. Combine all ingredients in blender and blend for three minutes on high. Pour into bowl. Cover with cheesecloth. Secure with rubber band. Place in a warm place with good air circulation for 6 hours. Remove cloth. Scrape off top oxidized layer and discard. Spoon middle layer into a seed bag. Hang bag in refrigerator overnight with a bowl underneath it to catch liquid. In the morning you will have seed cheese. Season with herbs and spices of choice. It will keep in the refrigerator up to 5 days. Eat 3-5 tablespoons daily. Great for digestion!

SOUPS

Delicious soups are a huge part of a live food diet. Eat them fresh. Soups are great for a quick nutritious meal.

Energy Soup (2 cups)

2 leaves romaine lettuce
4 leaves dark green kale
1 zucchini squash
½ avocado
1 cucumber
1 cup sprouts of choice
2 tablespoons dulse flakes
3/4 cup Rejuvelac or water

Cut up vegetables. Place ingredients in blender. Blend until smooth and creamy. Taste. Add additional seasonings to suit your taste. Serve immediately. Try to eat energy soup everyday for good balanced nutrition. Try different variations using different vegetables and leafy greens.

Spinach Avocado Soup - (6 servings)

5 cups filtered water
2 cups spinach
½ avocado
1 cup soaked cashews
1 teaspoon garlic powder
1 teaspoon onion powder
1 teaspoon Celtic sea salt

Blend all ingredients in blender until smooth and creamy. Taste. Adjust flavors as needed. Serve.

Health Journey

Emperor's Stew (8 servings)

2 quarts filtered hot water
2 cups shredded napa cabbage
1 cup sprouted barley or quinoa
1 cup chopped broccoli
1 cup chopped scallions
½ cup shredded carrots
½ cup soaked wakame
½ cup snow peas
¼ cup nama shoyu
¼ cup chopped cilantro
2 tablespoons sesame oil
½ teaspoon cayenne pepper (optional)

Combine all ingredients in a large bowl. Mix well.

Curry Vegetable Stew (8 servings)

1 chopped eggplant
2 cups chopped yellow squash
2 cups diced tomatoes
2 cups chopped spinach
2 quarts filtered hot water
2 cloves minced garlic
3 tablespoons mild curry powder
2 tablespoons nama shoyu
1 tablespoon cumin powder
½ teaspoon cayenne pepper
½ teaspoon chili powder
¼ cup lime juice
Celtic sea salt to taste
Agave nectar to taste

In large bowl or crock, place chopped vegetables. Add water and seasonings. Mix well. Taste. Adjust flavors.

SALADS

Veggie Kraut and sprouts add a new dimension to health and variety. Crunchy bean sprouts, flavorful broccoli sprouts, and spicy radish sprouts are great on salads.

Veggie Kraut (1 quart)

1 green cabbage
4 carrots
1 cup wakame
1 tablespoon apple cider vinegar
Juice from 1½ limes
1 teaspoon Celtic sea salt

Soak wakame with just enough water to cover. Remove outside leaves of cabbage and save. Chop cabbage. Shred carrots in food processor. Place all ingredients, including soak water, into large bowl or crock. Mix well with hands and pack it tightly. Cover with outside cabbage leaves. Place large plate and weight on top. Leave at room temperature for 2 days or until it is sour enough for your taste. Store in covered glass jar in refrigerator. Keeps up to 3 weeks.

Simple Salad (4 servings)

1 head chopped romaine lettuce
2 heads chopped kale
1 red onion sliced thinly
1/2 cup pitted black olives
2-3 tablespoons olive oil
Dash Celtic salt

Combine ingredients in bowl. Massage well with hands. Top with simple salad dressing on page 121.

Health Journey

Avocado Salad (4 servings)

1 head leafy green lettuce
1 head romaine lettuce
1 sliced red onion
1 sliced cucumber
2 sliced avocados
2 large chopped tomatoes
1 cup sunflower sprouts (or sprouts of choice)

Wash and chop lettuce. In large bowl, add all ingredients. Toss well.

Quinoa Salad (4 servings) *Complete Protein!*

2 cups sprouted quinoa
1 bunch washed and cut arugula
1 bunch washed and cut red leafy lettuce
1 sliced red onion
1 julienned red bell pepper
1 sliced yellow squash
1 sliced zucchini squash
½ sliced medium eggplant
½ cup walnut oil
¼ cup fresh lemon juice
1 tablespoon dried basil
1 tablespoon dried tarragon, dill or thyme
⅛ cup nama shoyu

In bowl, marinate yellow squash, zucchini, and eggplant with oil, lemon juice, basil, tarragon and nama shoyu for 1 hour. In large bowl, combine arugula, red leafy lettuce, quinoa, red onion, and red bell pepper. Mix well. Top with marinated vegetables. Serve immediately.

Sea Vegetable Salad (8 servings)

Sea vegetables are high in minerals and vitamins and have proven useful in healing high blood pressure, high cholesterol, anemia, and poor digestion. Good brands are Eden, Emerald Cove and Mitoku. Always begin by soaking for 20 minutes and straining. Save soak water for use in soups or for soaking seeds in.

Arame is high in protein, potassium, iron, calcium, iodine and Vitamins A, B1, B2.

Hijiki is very high in calcium, phosphorus, iron, protein and Vitamins A, B1, B2.

Wakame is high in protein, iron, calcium, magnesium Vitamins A, C, B1, B2, B12, Niacin.

1 head chopped green cabbage
½ cup soaked arame
½ cup soaked hijiki
½ cup soaked wakame
3 large finely chopped carrots
1 finely chopped red onion
1 diced red bell pepper
1 cup pine nut mayonnaise (see recipe on page 122)

Combine all ingredients in large bowl. Mix well. Serve immediately or refrigerate.

Health Journey

Ms. Lillian's Down Home Greens (4 servings)

These greens get better with time, so make enough for a few days. You won't miss the cooked version.

4 bunches collard greens
4 bunches kale or mustard greens
Flax oil to coat greens
2 large diced garlic cloves
1 diced sweet onion
Juice from 1 lemon
1 tablespoon apple cider vinegar
2 tablespoons agave nectar
1 tablespoon chili powder
2 tablespoons cumin powder
1 tablespoon Celtic sea salt
1 teaspoon cayenne powder
10 sliced Shitake mushrooms

Wash and cut greens removing stem. Coat greens with oil. Add seasonings. Mix well with hands. Taste. Adjust flavors. Add mushrooms. Let marinate overnight in refrigerator.

Sprout Salad (4 servings)

2 cups crunchy sprouts (adzuki, mung, and lentil)
2 heads leafy green lettuce
2 shredded carrots
2 seeded and diced tomatoes
4 diced scallions
¼ cup chopped cilantro
1 tablespoon lime juice
2 tablespoons hemp oil

Combine vegetables in a bowl. Add hemp oil and lime juice. Mix well. Serve immediately.

Recipes

SALAD DRESSINGS

Avocado Dressing (2 cups)

1 cup olive oil
1 peeled and chopped avocado
Juice from 3 limes
2 tablespoons agave nectar
2 cloves garlic
Dash sea salt

Blend all ingredients until smooth. Add water as needed.

Carrot Ginger Dressing (1 cup)

2 carrots
¼ cup coconut oil
1 tablespoon chopped ginger
½ cup filtered water
3 tablespoons agave nectar
1 tablespoon dried tarragon
 Nama shoyu to taste

Blend all ingredients until smooth.

Simple Salad Dressing (3/4 cup)

½ cup orange juice
2 tablespoons almond butter
1 clove garlic
3 tablespoons olive oil
4-6 dates
Nama shoyu or Celtic salt to taste

Blend all ingredients until smooth. Pour over simple salad.

Health Journey

Tahini Dressing (1½ cups)

1 cup soaked sesame seeds
⅛ cup lemon juice
¼ cup sesame oil
¼ cup filtered water
2 cloves garlic
1 tablespoon agave nectar
1 teaspoon Celtic sea salt
1 teaspoon nama shoyu

Combine all ingredients in blender. Blend until smooth.

Herb Vinaigrette Dressing (2 cups)

1 cup walnut oil
¼ cup apple cider vinegar
2 fresh basil leaves
1 clove garlic
½ teaspoon dried thyme
½ teaspoon onion powder
½ teaspoon Celtic sea salt

Blend all ingredients until smooth.

Pine Nut Mayonnaise (1-½ cups)

1 cup hemp or flax oil
1½ cups pine nuts, soaked and strained
⅛ cup lemon juice
2 tablespoons agave nectar
2 tablespoons dried tarragon
1 tablespoon dried parsley
1 teaspoon Celtic sea salt

In blender, combine all ingredients. Blend until creamy.

PÂTÉS

Pâtés are excellent by themselves, added to salads, served on crackers, stuffed inside a collard or lettuce leaf, or in a nori sheet.

Mock Salmon Pâté (1 quart)

3 cups macadamia nuts, soaked 8 hours and strained
3-4 finely chopped medium carrots
3 finely chopped scallions
2 finely chopped celery stalks
1 tablespoon Celtic sea salt
2 tablespoons kelp granules
Water as needed

In food processor, blend macadamia nuts and carrots until smooth, adding water as needed. Move to bowl. Add remaining ingredients. Mix well. Serve in a nori sheet or butter lettuce.

Mock Salmon Croquettes (6)

Mold pate into 3" croquettes. Top with ground pistachio nuts. Place on teflex sheet and dehydrate for 8 hours.

Curry Pâté (1 quart)

4 cups soaked walnuts
1 chopped medium zucchini
1½ tablespoons curry powder
2 tablespoons agave
Celtic sea salt to taste
Water as needed

In food processor, blend all ingredients until smooth.

Sea Vegetable Pâté (1 quart)

2 cups soaked macadamia nuts
1 cup sprouted sunflower seeds
2 chopped celery stalks
1 carrot chopped
¼ cup soaked wakame
¼ cup soaked arame
2 tablespoons soaked hijiki
Celtic sea salt to taste
Water as needed

In food processor, blend all ingredients, adding water as needed. Sprinkle with dulse flakes. Taste. Adjust flavors.

Pumpkin Seed Pâté (1 quart)

3 cups sprouted pumpkin seeds
1 chopped zucchini
1 chopped red bell pepper
5 soaked sun-dried tomatoes
1 tablespoon agave nectar (optional)
1 teaspoon kelp powder
1 teaspoon Celtic sea salt
Juice from 1 lime
Water as needed

In food processor, blend all ingredients, adding water as needed. Taste. Adjust flavors.

Collard Wraps

Soak collard leaves in warm water with a pinch of Celtic sea salt for 1 hour. Rinse and dry leaves. Trim vein. Spread pâté of choice across the bottom of leaf and top with sprouts. Fold ends, and roll.

SIDE DISHES

Sweet Basil Pilaf - (6 servings)

4 cups sprouted barley (or grain of choice)
2 sprigs basil (about 30-40 leaves)
1 handful spinach
1 chopped small sweet onion (Vidalia or Spanish)
1 large clove garlic
1 cup pine nuts
1 tablespoon Celtic sea salt
½ cup olive oil

Strain barley and place in bowl. Add onion. In blender, combine pine nuts, olive oil, spinach, basil, garlic and sea salt. Blend until creamy. Add to bowl and mix well.

Succotash (4 servings)

3 cups fresh corn cut off cob
3 cups diced okra or zucchini
3 cups diced tomatoes
1 diced onion
1 diced jalapeno pepper
2 cloves garlic
¼ cup lemon juice
1 tablespoon salt free Spike
1 tablespoon paprika
2 teaspoons cumin powder
1 teaspoon curry powder

In large bowl combine all ingredients. Mix well with hands. Let marinate in refrigerator for a few hours. If using okra, add just before serving.

Health Journey

Lip-Smacking Yams (4 servings)

3 small yams, peeled and cut in chunks
¼ cup dates, soaked 20 minutes and pitted
¼ cup raisins, soaked 20 minutes and strained
¼ cup pine nuts
¼ cup fresh orange juice
1 teaspoon cinnamon
½ teaspoon allspice
½ teaspoon nutmeg

Place yams, dates, raisins, pine nuts and orange juice in food processor and blend to a coarse consistency, adding more orange juice as needed. Transfer the mixture to a bowl and add seasonings. Mix well.

Jicama Potato Salad (4-8 servings)

Jicama (hee-kah-mah) looks like a large radish and is high in vitamin C, and has the texture of a potato, but less starchy and is sweet like a pear or apple.

1 large peeled and chopped jicama
1 cup sweet peas
½ cup pickles (cornichon or pickle of choice)
2 finely diced celery stalks
Celtic sea salt to taste
½ cup pine nuts
½ cup olive oil or oil of choice
1 tablespoon turmeric
1 teaspoon Celtic sea salt

In large bowl combine jicama, sweet peas, pickles, celery, and sea salt. In blender, blend remaining ingredients until creamy. Add to bowl. Mix well. Refrigerate and serve.

Recipes

Cajun Stuffing

This is the perfect side dish for the holidays or everyday!

2 cups soaked walnuts
4 cups sprouted sunflower seeds
1 large finely diced red bell pepper
1 large finely diced onion
1 large finely diced portabella mushroom
1 finely diced leek
2 finely diced celery stalks
⅛ cup olive oil
1 tablespoon garlic powder
1 tablespoon onion powder
1 tablespoon nama shoyu
2 tablespoons sage
1½ tablespoons poultry seasoning
1 tablespoon Cajun seasoning
1 tablespoon dried oregano
1 tablespoon dried thyme
1 tablespoon cumin
⅛ teaspoon cayenne pepper
1 teaspoon Celtic sea salt

In small bowl, combine bell pepper, onion, mushroom, leek, celery, olive oil, garlic powder, onion powder and nama shoyu. Mix well and set aside.

In food processor, pulse walnuts and sunflower seeds. Place in a large mixing bowl. Add remaining seasonings. Add vegetables and mix well. Taste and adjust flavors. Place on teflex sheet. Dehydrate 110°F until brown on top and moist inside, about 2 hours.

Serve warm. Refrigerate up to 3 days.

Health Journey

MAIN DISHES

Au Gratin Vegetables (4 servings)

2 heads chopped broccoli florets
1 chopped cauliflower
1 cup cubed portabella mushrooms
1 diced zucchini squash
1 diced yellow squash
1 diced red bell pepper
1 chopped sweet onion
2 cups soaked cashews
3 tablespoons lemon juice
2 tablespoons nutritional yeast
1 tablespoon miso paste
1 teaspoon Celtic sea salt
Water as needed

In a large bowl, combine the vegetables. Set aside. In blender, blend the remaining ingredients. Pour sauce over vegetables. Mix well. Let marinate overnight or place on teflex sheet and dehydrate for l hour. Serve warm.

Temperature Talk: As with baking, the temperature inside the dehydrator may be lower than the thermostat and the temperature of food is generally lower than the temperature inside the dehydrator. Therefore, preheat the dehydrator to 140°F while preparing food so that the dehydrator is warm when you put food in it. Use a thermostat to test the inside temperature of the dehydrator and a thermometer to test the food temperature. Once the dehydrator is has reached the desired temperature inside, you can adjust the thermostat.

Recipes

Pesto Pasta (4 servings)

1 peeled butternut squash
1 large zucchini

Spiralize squash using Spirooli. Top with pesto sauce (see recipe on page 113).

Smothered Portabella Mushrooms *(4 servings)*

4 large portabella mushrooms
2 cups mushroom gravy (See recipe on page 112)

Place mushrooms top side down in casserole dish. Pour gravy over mushrooms. Spread generously with hands. Turn mushrooms top side up. Partially slice so gravy oozes in center of mushrooms. Let marinate for 30 minutes, or place on teflex sheet and dehydrate 110°F for 1 hour, basting with gravy. Serve warm.

Chili (4 servings)

4 diced zucchini squashes
4 finely diced carrots
2 diced red bell peppers
3 diced tomatoes
2 cups corn
1 diced onion
1 cup pitted black olives (optional)
2 cups chili sauce (see recipe page 113)

In large bowl combine all vegetables. Add 2 cups chili sauce. Mix well. Serve alone or over sprouted barley.

Health Journey

Walnut Patties (6 patties)

8 cups soaked walnuts
1½ cups soaked sun-dried tomatoes
2 cloves garlic
1 tablespoon cumin powder
1 tablespoon chili powder
1 teaspoon Celtic sea salt

Combine all ingredients in food processor, and pulse until ground. Form into 3" patties. Dehydrate at 110°F for 8 hours. Flip. Dehydrate until dry.

Hemp Falafel (25 balls)

2 cups soaked Brazil Nuts
2 cups soaked walnuts
2 cups sprouted sunflower seeds
1 cup hemp nuts
2 tablespoons tahini
3 tablespoons minced garlic
3 tablespoons fresh lemon juice
3 tablespoons curry powder
3 tablespoons cumin powder
3 tablespoons chopped fresh parsley
2 tablespoons sesame oil
1 tablespoon celery powder
1 teaspoon chili powder
1 teaspoon coriander
Celtic sea salt to taste

In food processor, blend nuts, seeds, tahini, garlic and sea salt. Move to bowl. Add remaining ingredients. Mix well. Form batter into balls using an ice cream scoop and place on dehydrator sheet. Dehydrate for 8 hours at 110°F until crisp on the outside and moist inside. Serve warm. Refrigerate up to one week.

Tamale Pie (9" pie pan, 8-10 servings)

Nut Meat

2 cups soaked walnuts
1 tablespoon olive oil
½ tablespoon dried oregano
½ tablespoon paprika
½ tablespoon minced garlic
½ tablespoon apple cider vinegar
1 teaspoon Celtic sea salt
¼ teaspoon cayenne (optional)
Filtered water as needed

Pulse all ingredients in food processor until nuts are ground, adding water as needed. Taste and adjust flavors. Place nut meat in bottom of 9" glass pie pan patting in down evenly. Set aside

Chili

See recipe on page 129.

Top nut meat with chili.

Corn Bread Topping

3 cups oat flour
½ cup pine nuts
½ cup soaked cashews
2 cups fresh corn
¾ cup filtered water
1 teaspoon Celtic sea salt
1 teaspoon vanilla extract
3 tablespoons agave nectar

Health Journey

Place oat flour and 1 cup corn In large mixing bowl. Place remaining ingredients in blender. Blend to pancake batter consistency. Add to mixing bowl. Mix well with hands. Batter should be like dough, not too wet.

Place plastic wrap in a glass 9" pie pan. Put dough in the wrap pressing it down with your fingers to form size of the pan. Lift the plastic wrap and place corn bread on top of chili. Smooth edges using spatula.

Dehydrate for 25 minutes at 110°F. Serve immediately. Refrigerate up to 4 days.

Veggie Hash (4 servings)

1 cup sprouted buckwheat
1 cup soaked Brazil nuts
3 shredded carrots
1 chopped red onion
½ chopped red bell pepper
¼ cup fresh Italian parsley
2 garlic cloves
1 teaspoon chili powder
1 teaspoon paprika
1 teaspoon Celtic sea salt

Place buckwheat in bowl. In food processor, combine remaining ingredients. Pulse until mixed well, but still chunky. Add to bowl and mix well. Taste and adjust flavors. Serve immediately or warm in the dehydrator. Refrigerate up to 5 days.

Recipes

Broccoli Spinach Quiche (9" pie, 8-12 servings)

Crust

2 cups soaked and dehydrated walnuts
¼ cup raisins
1 tablespoon paprika
1 tablespoon onion powder
1 tablespoon garlic powder

In food processor, process all ingredients until uniformly fine. Press evenly into glass pie pan.

Filling

1 head chopped broccoli
2 cups chopped spinach
2 cups Rejuvelac
3 tablespoons psyllium powder
1 small chopped onion
1 cup soaked macadamia nuts
1 cup nutritional yeast
¼ cup lemon juice
1 tablespoon miso paste
¾ cup flax meal
1 tablespoon turmeric
¼ teaspoon cayenne
3 tablespoons agave nectar
1 teaspoon Celtic sea salt

Place spinach and broccoli in mixing bowl. In blender, blend macadamia nuts, Rejuvelac, lemon juice, miso, ½ cup nutritional yeast, cayenne and agave until creamy. Add more liquid if needed. Pour in mixing bowl. Add remaining ingredients to bowl. Mix well. Place filling in pie plate. Dehydrate for 1 hour at 110°F. Serve warm. Refrigerate up to 4 days.

BREAD, FRITTERS AND PANCAKES

Flax Bread (four 9" dehydrator trays)

2 cups flax meal
1 papaya
½ avocado
1 tablespoon cumin powder
1 tablespoon chili powder
1 tablespoon garlic powder
1 tablespoon onion powder
1 teaspoon Celtic sea salt
3 cups filtered water

In Vita-mix blender, blend all ingredients until smooth. Pour mixture onto dehydrator sheet. Spread evenly, making sure dough is not too thick in the middle. Dehydrate at 110°F for 6 hours. Flip onto mesh sheet and continue dehydrating until soft and dry. Cut into desired sizes. Store in zip lock bag in refrigerator.

Corn Fritters (36 fritters)

A great snack and comfort food!

See recipe for corn bread topping on page 131.

After batter is mixed, place dough onto mesh dehydrator tray using fingers. Do not handle dough too much by trying to form it into fritters. Simply pick it up and put it on the mesh dehydrator tray.

Dehydrate until dry, about 1 hour at 110°F. Serve warm. Refrigerate up to 5 days. Be careful not to eat too many.

Recipes

Blueberry Pancakes

1 cup oat flour
½ large papaya
1 teaspoon cinnamon
½ teaspoon Celtic sea salt
½ cup agave nectar
2 cups golden flax meal
1 teaspoon vanilla extract
Filtered water
2 cups fresh blueberries

Place oat flour in large mixing bowl. Place remaining ingredients, except water and blueberries in blender. Add water to 8 cup level. Blend until smooth. Add to bowl. Add blueberries. Mix well.

Using a ½ cup measuring cup, place 9 individual cups of batter onto teflex dehydrator sheet, 3 to a row. Moisten hands with water. Press each pancake into 1/4" pancakes. Dehydrate for 4 hours at 110°F. Flip. Dehydrate until pancakes are spongy, but not wet inside. Serve warm.

Pineapple Mango Syrup

¼ cup agave nectar
½ cup filtered water
¼ cup pineapple chunks
½ teaspoon vanilla extract
Pinch Celtic sea salt or nama shoyu

Place all ingredients in blender. Blend for 5 seconds. Pour over pancakes. Refrigerate up to 7 days.

Health Journey

DESSERTS

These delicious desserts are great for breakfast, lunch and dinner. Low in fat and calories, they are the perfect dessert and snack food. Be mindful of overeating!

Blueberry Mango Pie (9", 8-10 servings)

Crust

2 cup soaked and dehydrated walnuts
1 cup raisins
1 teaspoon nutmeg

In food processor, process all ingredients until uniformly fine. Spread evenly into glass pie pan.

Filling

1 pint fresh blueberries
2 thinly sliced mangoes
12-14 pitted dates

Layer thinly sliced mango on top of crust. Blend half the blueberries with 6 dates until smooth. Pour evenly over mangoes using spatula. Layer remainder of sliced mangoes. Blend remaining half of blueberries with 6 dates. Pour evenly over mangoes using spatula.

Let chill for 45 minutes to 1 hour.

Recipes

Papaya Delight (6 servings)

1 large papaya
2 mangoes
1 pint fresh raspberries
6 pitted dates

Cut the papaya in half the long way. Place the seeds in a bowl and set aside. Peel the papaya and chop into chunks. Place in blender. Peel the mangoes, cut fruit from around the pit and add to blender. Add raspberries and dates.

Blend all ingredients until smooth. It will have a thick pudding consistency. Using an ice cream scoop serve in bowl. Garnish with a few papaya seeds.

Nutty Butter Brownie (9", 8-10 servings)

12 cups soaked walnuts
1 package dried figs (about 8)
1 cup raw carob powder
½ cup agave nectar
1 cup raw almond butter

In food processor, combine walnuts, figs and carob powder. Blend to fine meal. Add ¼ cup agave to make sticky. Move ¾ of mixture to spring form pan and form into shape of shallow bowl. Add ½ cup almond butter. Spread. Add remaining ¼ of mixture. Spread. Set aside.

In blender, blend remaining agave and almond butter. Drizzle over brownie. Serve immediately.

Berry Cheesecake (9", 12-16 servings)

Crust

2 cups soaked and dehydrated walnuts
1 cup raisins
1 teaspoon nutmeg

In food processor, process ingredients until they are uniformly fine. Cover bottom of spring form pan with plastic wrap. Press mixture into pan. Set aside.

Filling

4 cups macadamia nuts, soaked and strained
1½ cups coconut oil
1 cup mixed berries
1 cup agave nectar
¾ cup lemon juice
¾ cup filtered water
4 tablespoons psyllium powder
2 teaspoons vanilla extract
½ teaspoon Celtic sea salt

Combine all ingredients in blender. Blend until smooth, adding water as needed. Pour on top of crust. Freeze for 20 minutes.

Topping

½ cup mixed berries
12 pitted dates, soaked 1 hour

Strain dates, and place in blender with berries. Blend until smooth. Once cheesecake is set, spread on top of cheesecake. Freeze for 1 hour. Serve.

Recipes

Coconut Cake (9", 12-16 servings)

9 cups oat flour (ground oat groats or rolled oats)
2 cups chopped pecans (soaked, strained, dehydrated)
3 cups unsweetened shredded coconut
1½ cups agave nectar
1 level tablespoon ground cloves
Water as needed (about 2 cups)
½ pineapple pulsed in food processor

In large bowl, combine oat flour, nuts, coconut, pineapple, cloves and agave nectar. Mix well. Add water while kneading the mixture. The batter should be moist but not runny. If too much water is added let stand for 15-20 minutes. Form dough into two large balls. Press each dough ball into a spring form pan.

Icing

6 cups unsweetened shredded coconut
1 cup coconut meat (from young Thai coconut)
4 cups filtered water
1 cup agave nectar
¼ cup lemon juice
1 vanilla bean or 2 tablespoons vanilla extract
3 tablespoons psyllium powder

Blend 4 cups shredded coconut, and remaining ingredients in high-speed blender until creamy. If too watery add a little more shredded coconut.

Remove 1 cake from spring form pan and place on a plate (this is your bottom layer). Spread Icing on top of this layer of cake. Remove other cake from spring form pan and place on top of bottom layer. Ice the top layer of cake, spreading icing along the sides of cake. Top with shredded coconut.

Health Journey

Mixed Berry Fruit Parfait (four 2-cup servings)

This dessert is perfect for breakfast. Omit the fruit jelly and add fresh fruit instead. Or just have the granola with nut milk! Granola also makes a great snack on its own.

The cream is perfect over fruit or added to smoothies instead of yogurt.

Granola

4 cups rolled oats
1 cup sprouted buckwheat
2 cups soaked and dehydrated chopped walnuts
1 teaspoon cloves
1 teaspoon cinnamon
1 teaspoon allspice
¼ cup agave nectar
¼ cup filtered water
½ teaspoon Celtic sea salt

Mix all ingredients in large bowl. Place on mesh dehydrator tray. Dehydrate at 110°F until crunchy and chewy.

Fruit Jelly

1 cup each blueberries, raspberries, strawberries
2 cups filtered water
¼ cup agave nectar
2 tablespoons lemon juice
2 tablespoons psyllium powder

In blender, blend all ingredients until smooth. Set aside.

Macadamia Nut Cream

2 cups soaked macadamia nuts
2 cups filtered water
Meat from one young Thai coconut
¼ cup fresh orange juice
¼ teaspoon vanilla extract
6 pitted dates

In blender, blend all ingredients until smooth. Set aside.

In parfait or wine glass layer granola, jelly, and cream. Repeat. Top with granola sprinkles. Serve immediately or chilled. Granola will keep in zip lock bag indefinitely. Jelly and Cream will keep in refrigerator up to 5 days.

Vanilla Bean Ice Cream (12 servings)

4 cups soaked cashews
Meat from 2 young Thai coconuts
1 cup coconut oil
1 cup agave nectar
2 vanilla beans
1 tablespoon coarse Celtic sea salt
Filtered water

In Vita-mix blender, combine cashews, coconut meat, coconut oil, agave, vanilla beans, and sea salt. Add water to fill container to 8 cups. Blend well until smooth and creamy using tamper to stir. Pour into shallow stainless steel bowl. Freeze until firm. Will keep up to 2 weeks in the freezer.

To make different flavors, add desired fruit or flavorings before blending.

Health Journey

RECOMMENDATIONS FOR BETTER HEALTH

1. Sprout wheat berries, quinoa, barley, or buckwheat to make Rejuvelac. See sprouting instructions on page 105. Sprout enough seeds or grains to make 2 batches of Rejuvelac.

2. Purchase two wide-mouth glass gallon jars. These can be found at the Container Store.

3. When seeds are sprouted, prepare Rejuvelac according to recipe on page 108.

4. Once you strain the Rejuvelac, start another batch.

5. Drink at least two glasses of Rejuvelac daily.

6. Prepare seed cheese and energy soup using Rejuvelac, and eat regularly.

7. Make Rejuvelac, seed cheese, and energy soup your diet staples. You will notice an improvement in your energy level, digestion, and elimination.

8. If you haven't eliminated animal products from your diet, decrease by half the amount of animal products you consume. Eat smaller portions or decrease the number of days that you eat animal products.

9. Eat a fresh salad with sprouts daily. Always add sprouts to your salads for protein!

7

LIFESTYLE

Obtaining optimal health means making lifestyle changes in addition to dietary changes. Gone are the days when you could party, drink and drug without consequence. Leading this type of lifestyle eventually takes its toll on you and leads to premature aging, illness and disease--all of the conditions we want to avoid.

Instead, we want to adopt a lifestyle that keeps us looking and feeling good for as long as possible. Vanity is a great motivator because it will make you do the things you may not want to do for the sake of looking good. That's a good start, but it will take more than vanity to maintain a healthy lifestyle for the rest of your life. You need to develop an appreciation for the things that will lead you to the path of self fulfillment. When you attain self fulfillment, you will see beauty quite differently than the physical beauty apparent in our youth. You will begin to see beauty in everything and everyone. This is a worthy goal. While diet plays an important role in obtaining enlightenment, there are many other factors that are equally important.

A POSITIVE ATTITUDE toward life will attract positive results. A positive attitude reflects everything you do and everything that happens to you. It determines how you deal with situations, outcomes of those situations, and people's response to you. Vibrations of your conscious and unconscious thoughts and desires have the power to manifest. A desire triggers a thought; a thought creates an action, actions create destiny. Thoughts of love, hatred, happiness, anger, lust, jealousy, compassion and revenge leave an imprint on our body, emotions and spirit. Negative thoughts can make us ill just as positive thoughts can make us heal.

Try to see the positive in each situation and person you encounter including yourself. Focus on the good things in your life—the things that are working. Build a strong foundation from there.

Replace negative thoughts with positive thoughts. Use affirmations to reinforce your positive attitude. An affirmation is something true about you that is positive, such as "I am a good person," "I am smart," "I am strong," "I am forgiving," "I am patient," you get the picture. Begin by making a list of things that you like about yourself. Whenever someone pays you a compliment, add it to the list. Ask your close friends and relatives to tell you some of the things they admire about you. It is sometimes difficult for us to see qualities we have that others see. Say these affirmations to yourself at least twice a day and as often as necessary. If you are having a stressful day, take some deep breaths and say your affirmations.

Create positive thoughts through the practice of good deeds such as holding the elevator for someone or helping your neighbor with her groceries or giving up your seat for someone on the bus or train.

BREATHING is essential to life. The deeper the breath, the more oxygen our bodies receive. Illness and disease cannot take hold in an oxygenated body. Is there a right and a wrong way to breathe? Let's just say there's a good and better way to breathe. Most of us take shallow breaths and do not take in enough

Lifestyle

oxygen. We breathe deeply when we yawn. Just hearing the word yawn makes you yawn! We yawn to get more oxygen in our body. Notice what happens when you yawn. Your diaphragm expands, the jaw opens wide, the lungs fill up, and the ribcage and spine lift. When you yawn, you are taking a deep involuntary breath. Practice yawning. Make yourself yawn right now, if you haven't already. How do you feel? Are you more relaxed? Begin to be more conscious of your breathing. Focus on the exhalation, to get rid of carbon dioxide, and inhale to bring oxygen to the blood. Practice this simple exercise daily. Inhale deeply. Hold your breath for 10 seconds, and then exhale slowly and completely. Repeat. By holding the breath you are allowing the breathing to slow down and more oxygen to enter the lungs and respiratory system.

RELAXATION. Deep breathing promotes relaxation. I may not have much time to relax, but I go through my day in a relaxed manner. The more relaxed I am, the happier I am. That's not to say that taking time out to relax is not important. It is important, but it seems we must find time in our busy schedules to relax. Pick times out of your day when you can relax. Lunch time is a good time. Instead of eating a large lunch, eat a small one and allow time to put your feet up, and take some deep breaths. This will rejuvenate you, and you will have plenty of energy to complete your day without getting that afternoon drop in energy. When you feel tired, take some deep breaths.

Usually it is the things we enjoy doing that bring about relaxation, like listening to music, cooking, laughing, or reading a good book. Relaxation techniques include yoga, visualization, massage and meditation.

Health Journey

SLEEP. I find it best to have a routine when it comes to getting a good night's sleep. Go to bed and arise at the same time each day. Allow enough time for a restful, recuperative sleep. This may mean going to bed earlier to get a full 8 hours of sleep. Create a relaxing sleep environment. A comfortable bed with fresh linen is essential. Perhaps you want to open a window to create good air flow. Remove the television and related electronics from the room that you sleep in. Make sure the room is dark enough—close the shades and curtains. Place noisy clocks away from earshot.

The more relaxed you are at the end of the day, the better you will sleep. Try meditating to relax your mind. Take a hot bath before bedtime while listening to soothing music. Try not to eat within two hours of bedtime. Absolutely no alcohol, nicotine or caffeine close to bedtime. Drink water or herbal tea instead. Avoid watching television before bed, particularly scary movies. Read a book. Give yourself a massage.

If you suffer from insomnia, in addition to the above suggestions, put a few drops of the essential oil of lavender on your pillowcase before sleeping, or put a drop of Celtic sea salt on your tongue to relax you. Clear your head by writing down your thoughts. If that doesn't work, get up and do something productive.

Love yourself as you would your child. This means nurturing yourself.

MEDITATION. Concentration of mind is absolutely necessary for spiritual success. It is concentration and meditation that eventually lead to the realization of the Self. Meditation is keeping up an increasing flow of God-consciousness. All worldly thoughts are shut out from the mind. It is filled or saturated with divine

Lifestyle

presence. Meditation is the seventh rung or step on the ladder of Yoga. Forget the body and surroundings. Forgetting is the highest spiritual practice. It helps meditation a great deal and makes the approach to God easier. By remembering God, you can forget everything else.

To meditate, sit in a quiet place in a cross-legged position (Lotus). Repeat a bible verse or hymn in your mind for ten minutes. This will elevate the mind. Then stop this kind of thinking and fix the mind on one idea. Do not think of anything else. Do not allow any worldly thoughts to enter the mind. Do not allow it to think of any physical or mental enjoyment. When it indulges in these thoughts, bring it back to the one idea. Gently allow divine thoughts to flow.

Meditation is helpful in regulating your emotions and moods, for it develops strong and pure thoughts. Regular meditation opens the avenues of intuitive knowledge, makes the mind calm and steady, awakens an ecstatic feeling and brings the student of Yoga in contact with the Supreme Spirit.

Begin by meditating for half an hour in the early hours of the morning, and you will be able to work peacefully throughout the day. Nothing will disturb your mind.

EXERCISE activates the sweat glands and allows built-up toxins to be released through the skin. Furthermore, it is an excellent method of mentally detoxifying. Not only will you have more energy and feel better, but you will have fun in the process.

As we age our metabolism drops by 2% every decade, thereby decreasing lean muscle and increasing fat. Designing a diet and exercise regime to balance nature is the best defense. Having a positive attitude about fitness will help you to accept the fact that you must include physical activity at all ages of life. Here are some suggestions from fitness gurus:

In our 20s we need weight training to develop muscle definition and bone density crucial for staying active and preventing osteoporosis later in life. Cardio three times a week is also important, and includes dancing, fast walking, kickboxing, spinning, swimming, and aerobics.

In our 30s we have to work harder to stay fit. That means stepping up your workout. Include circuit training (cardio and resistance) three times per week and high intensity cardio once a week. The fitness level you set up in your 30s will determine what your body will look like going forward. This is the time to be serious and consistent.

In our 40s is when we begin to bulge in the torso, belly and back. You will need one hour of weight training 3 days a week, and 45 minutes of low intensity cardio 5 days a week to battle the bulge.

In our 50s loss of muscle mass and tone, as well as belly fat, begin to show. Stretching and toning is imperative in addition to low intensity cardio four to six days a week, and weight training twice a week.

In our 60s we begin to develop aches and pains and you may need to push yourself physically a little harder. Challenging cardio such as fast walking or swimming three days a week is good, plus three days of light, slow weight.

Lifestyle

Cardio and weight training doesn't have to mean joining a gym. There are many choices such as swimming, African dance, belly dance, jazz dance, tap dance, jogging, fast walking, cycling, roller skating, jumping rope, and climbing stairs. Keep an open mind and try new things. Perhaps there's a sport you have always wanted to play. Now's a good time to start!

Rebounding develops balance, coordination, rhythm, timing, dexterity and kinesthetic awareness. It exercises the body at the cellular level. You're not just exercising the muscles, you're also exercising the skeleton. As a result, rebounding has proven effective in building bone mass and preventing osteoporosis.

Qigong (Chee gung) is the art and science of personal cultivation to promote health, longevity and self-sufficiency. It offers a variety of exercises including physical movement balanced with quiet and direct contemplation. With regular practice, Qigong will benefit internal organs as well as external muscles, joints and extremities. Qigong will enhance your immune, digestive, respiratory and circulatory systems. It improves balance, strength and stamina, and will enhance your self awareness, vitality and personal power.

If you are just starting to exercise, begin by stretching, toning and walking. Take yoga, body conditioning or Pilates™ classes, and walk 30 minutes a day. There are also many excellent exercise video tapes and DVDs on the above subjects. Exercising at home requires a great deal of motivation. Perhaps you have a friend or relative that you can exercise with. Select someone who is motivated. Set attainable goals, and reward yourself with a spa treatment when you achieve those goals.

Health Journey

RECOMMENDATIONS FOR BETTER HEALTH

1. Upon rising every morning, give your body a good stretch.

2. Practice breathing exercises and yawning daily.

3. Take a meditation class, or join a meditation group.

4. Count your blessings. Give thanks for the many blessings you receive daily.

5. Acknowledge the things you like and admire about yourself. Look in the mirror and say to yourself out loud, "I love myself because...."

6. Make a list of all the things you are grateful for.

7. Visualize the things you want in life.

8. Exercise at least 5 times per week and include cardio and weight training. Work with a personal trainer to get you started.

9. Trust your body's unlimited healing capabilities.

10. Cancel negative thinking and negative people.

11. Practice the 5 Ps: Purpose, Positive Attitude, Patience, Persistence and Prayer.

12. Sit or walk in the sunlight everyday if possible.

13. Laugh, cry, play and enjoy life. Don't be afraid to feel!

BIBLIOGRAPHY AND RECOMMENDED READING

1. "The Importance of Good Nutrition, Herbs & Phytochemicals," Getty T. Ambau, Falcon Press.

2. "Structured Healing," Harold Magoun Jr., D.O., F.A.A.O., self published by author.

3. "Good Carbs, Bad Carbs," Johanna Burani, M.D., R.D., C.D.E., and Linda Rao, M.Ed., Marlow & Company.

4. "The Complete Idiot's Guide to Looking and Feeling Younger," Sallie Batson and Hattie, Alpha Books.

5. Earl Mindell's Vitamin Bible for the 21st Century," Earl Mindell, Warner Books.

6. "Eight Weeks To Optimum Health," Andrew Weil, M.D., Alfred A. Knoff.

7. "Drugs Masquerading as Foods," Suzar.

8. "The Natural Way to Vibrant Health," Norman W. Walker, Ph.D., Norwalk Press.

9. "Dr. Mercola's Total Health," Joseph Mercola, M.D., Mercola.com.

10. "The Life Food Recipe Book," Annie & David Jubb, self published by authors.

11. "The Breast Cancer Prevention Plan," Edward J. Conley, Ph.D., McGraw-Hill.

12. "Soy Alert," The Weston A. Price Foundation, Wise Traditions.

13. "Rainbow Green Live-Food Cuisine," Gabriel Cousens, M.D., North Atlantic Books.

14. "Your Body's Many Cries For Water," F. Batmanghelidj, M.D., Global Health Solutions, Inc.

15. "Water & Salt, The Essence of Life," Dr. Med. Barbara Hendel, Peter Ferreira, self published.

16. "Eating for Beauty," David Wolfe, Maul Brothers Publishing.

17. "Goddesses & Angels," Doreen Virtue, Ph.D., Hay House, Inc.

18. "Seeds of Deception," Jeffrey M. Smith, Yes Books.

19. "The Cure for All Diseases," Hulda Regehr Clark, Ph.D., N.D., New Century Press.

20. "Constipation is a Serious Health Concern," Renew Life.

21. "African Holistic Health," Dr. Llaila O. Afrika, A&B Publishers Group.

22. "Sproutman's Kitchen Garden Cookbook," Steve Meyerowitz, Sproutman Publications.

AFTERWARD

We have learned so much in writing this book. It has strengthened our commitment to achieving optimal health, vitality and longevity.

We offer these words of encouragement. Focus on the positive things in your life, and live in the present. Yesterday is gone, and tomorrow is yet to come. Don't let the beauty of the moment pass while thinking about the past or future. Be fully present. This requires a great deal of listening. Learn to listen completely. A fun way to practice listening is to repeat someone's name in your head when being introduced. See if you can remember everyone's name. Try to remember something about that person that makes them unique, their hair, eyes, nose, or clothing.

Try to see and experience people and things as they are, without judgment. Our judgments are based on our thoughts and experiences, and have no relevance or truth. Rely on your intuition to guide you in dealing with people and situations.

Be truthful with yourself and others. The whole truth and nothing but. Telling the truth will clear your conscience, relax your mind, and elevate your thinking.

Only then can you begin to focus on things that are important in your life. Honesty is the foundation to building strong relationships based on truth and mutual respect.

Be fearless. It's the only way to get what you want. Face your fear and it will vanish. The mind deceives us through imaginary fears. Learn to cogitate, discriminate, reflect and meditate, and your fear will be transformed into faith and confidence. Be courageous and patient in the face of obstacles. Let your actions speak for your heart.

Never give up! Life can take us to some unexpected places. Knowing and loving yourself helps you to see the positive side of each situation and respond accordingly. This requires a great deal of surrender and trust. Accepting that you are powerless eliminates worry.

Life is a beautiful journey, and being healthy and vibrant is the best way to enjoy life at any age. When you live a healthy life you become ageless, because you are free from illness and disease, you have powerful positive thoughts and you only attract good things to you. This is the kind of life I want to live, how about you?

"The secret of happiness, you see, is not found in seeking more, but in developing the capacity to enjoy less."

Dan Millman, Way of Peaceful Warrior

Book Order Form

Online orders: www.rawsoul.com
Email: rawsoul@rawsoul.com

Postal orders:
Mail this form to Raw Soul
348 W. 145th Street, New York, NY 10039
Phone: (212) 491-5859

1-11 books $21.95 each
12 or more $13.00 each

Quantity   **Amount**
_____ $_____

U.S. Shipping and Handling $4.50 for 1st book $_____
$1.65 for each additional book. $_____

International Shipping and Handling $9.00 $_____
for first book, $5 each additional book $_____

                                          Sub-Total $_____

                                              Total $_____

Payment by Check or Money Order payable to Raw Soul

Name_____

Address_____

City_____ State_____

Country_____ Zip_____

Telephone_____

Email_____